Objective Questions
Orthopaedic Nursin

Elizabeth M. Evans SRN ONC RNT
Formerly Tutor at the Robert Jones and Agnes Hunt Orthopaedic Hospital, Oswestry, Shropshire

Foreword by
Mary Powell OBE SRN MCSP Orthopaedic Nursing Certificate
Formerly Matron, Robert Jones and Agnes Hunt Orthopaedic Hospital, Oswestry, Shropshire

CHURCHILL LIVINGSTONE
EDINBURGH LONDON MELBOURNE AND NEW YORK 1987

CHURCHILL LIVINGSTONE
Medical Division of Longman Group UK Limited

Distributed in the United States of America by Churchill Livingstone Inc., 1560 Broadway, New York, N.Y. 10036, and by associated companies, branches and representatives throughout the world.

First published 1987

ISBN 0 443 02473 1

British Library Cataloguing in Publication Data
Evans, Elizabeth M.
Objective questions in orthopaedic nursing.
1. Orthopedic nursing — Problems, exercises, etc.
I. Title
610.73'677 RD 753

Library of Congress Cataloging in Publication Data
Evans, Elizabeth M.
Objective questions in orthopaedic nursing.
Bibliography: p.
1. Orthopedic nursing — Examinations, questions, etc.
I. Title. [DNLM: 1. Orthopedics — nursing — examination questions. WY 18 E9250]
RD753.E83 1986 610.73'6 86–9559

Produced by Longman Singapore Publishers (Pte) Ltd.
Printed in Singapore

Objective Questions in Orthopaedic Nursing

To the memory of my father and mother who sadly died before seeing this book published.

Foreword

This book is designed as an aid to the nurse whose special study is the care of the orthopaedic patient. It will also be most helpful to those tutors in Schools of Nursing who must deal with this subject, and to nurses involved in in-service education in orthopaedic wards and departments. It will be useful not only in this country but also overseas.

The book deals with objective questions related to orthopaedics in a practical, lucid manner, and as well as being an aid to study it will help the nurse to apply the principles of the nursing process to the orthopaedic patient.

As one with a lifetime's interest in the subject, and who knew the author as a dedicated orthopaedic nurse and an excellent ward sister, it gives me great pleasure to write the foreword to this book. I am sure it will be a great success.

M.P.

Preface

When objective type questions were introduced into the final examination for the Orthopaedic Nursing Certificate it was clear to me that there were no books available for nurses studying orthopaedics to use for practice. The books which were on the market were either American, with their unfamiliar terminology, or geared towards students doing their general training and so did not cover the subject in sufficient depth. The aim of this book is to give nurses specialising in this subject practice with these types of questions, and so help them with learning and revision: they are not intended to simulate examination papers.

The book is written in two parts. The first part deals with anatomy and physiology, orthopaedic conditions and trauma, and nursing care, and is designed to test the student's previous knowledge. When going through the answers students should use a textbook for reference and further study so that they increase their knowledge rather than use the experience as yet another 'test'.

The second part of the book consists of nursing care studies with objective type questions related to each condition. When writing these care studies I have tried to cover many aspects of orthopaedic nursing including the assignment of patients to individual nurses, the assessment of the patient's needs, and the planning and evaluation of care following the nursing process. Questions cover anatomy and physiology, pathology, treatment and nursing care as they apply to the particular condition. I have attempted to write questions which test the student's knowledge of facts, principles, understanding and evaluation, and have written out the answers in full so that the student will see why I have selected a particular answer as being correct.

I would like to thank Mary Emmerson Law and Dinah Bagshaw of Churchill Livingstone for their help and encouragement in preparing this book and for editing it: also the publisher's artists for producing the illustrations.

To Mary Powell I should like to express my gratitude for her encouragement and enthusiasm, for writing the foreword and for allowing me to use her material and illustrations. My thanks also go to Churchill Livingstone for the use of illustrations from the work of the late Professor Sir John Charnley; to Mr Gwyn Evans and Faber for the photograph of a Pavlik harness; and to Miss Kathleen Nicoll for her helpful suggestions.

I am grateful to many members of staff of the Robert Jones and Agnes Hunt Orthopaedic Hospital for their help, in particular Miss J.W. Jones and the staff of the School of Nursing for their interest and suggestions; to the orthopaedic student nurses for trying out the case histories; to Barbara Woods and Alison Dixon for their help with the case history on congenital dislocation of the hip; to David and Joyce Jones for preparing the photographs; and to many others who have helped in many ways.

Finally, a special word of thanks must go to Llinos and Kathryn who looked after my little boy so that I was able to spend time on research and writing; and to my husband, Bryan, for his forbearance and for encouraging me to continue when family and farming commitments were heavy. Without their support this book would never have been written.

Oswestry, 1987 E.M.E.

Contents

Section One

Anatomy and physiology; orthopaedic conditions and trauma; orthopaedic nursing

Multiple choice questions *(Answers to Q. 1–42 appear on p. 47)*
The questions in this section are of the multiple choice type. Study each question and from the list of possible answers select the *one* which you think is correct.

---

1. Trabeculae are found in:
   A. Compact bone
   B. Cancellous bone
   C. The medullary cavity of long bones
   D. Children's bones only.

2. Bone-building cells are called:
   A. Osteoblasts
   B. Osteoclasts
   C. Osteophytes
   D. Osteocytes.

3. Which one of the following is a characteristic of a typical cervical vertebra?
   A. A foramen in the transverse process
   B. A small neural canal
   C. A long transverse process
   D. A hatchet-shaped spinous process.

4. The part of the sacrum which articulates with the ilium to form the sacroiliac joint is called the:
   A. Ala of the sacrum
   B. Auricular surface
   C. Tuberosity
   D. Superior facet.

5. The hamstring muscles:
   A. Adduct the hip
   B. Extend the knee
   C. Internally rotate the hip
   D. Flex the knee.

6. The branch of the lumbo-sacral plexus which supplies the adductor muscles of the hip is the:
   A. Sciatic nerve
   B. Femoral nerve
   C. Obturator nerve
   D. Genito-femoral nerve.

7. Which one of the following is the point of insertion of the triceps muscle?
   A. Coronoid process
   B. Coronoid fossa
   C. Radial tuberosity
   D. Olecranon process.

8. The ankle joint is formed by the:
   A. Tibia, fibula and talus
   B. Tibia and talus
   C. Tibia, fibula and navicular
   D. Talus and calcaneus.

9. Which of the following muscles abducts the hip joint?
   A. Semimembranosus
   B. Psoas
   C. Gluteus medius
   D. Iliacus.

10. In life the bones of the forearm are joined by the:
   A. Fascia lata
   B. Interosseus membrane
   C. Linea alba
   D. Flexor retinaculum.

11. The muscle spindle:
   A. Has sensory but no motor innervation
   B. Is associated with pain sensation
   C. Is involved in the maintenance of posture
   D. Is found in heart muscle only.

12. Which of the following hormones controls the blood calcium level?
    A. Thyroxin
    B. Cortisone
    C. Parathormone
    D. Growth hormone.

13. Which of the following vitamins is necessary for the absorption of calcium?
    A. Vitamin A
    B. Vitamin C
    C. Vitamin B_{12}
    D. Vitamin D.

14. The symphysis pubis is an example of a:
    A. Synovial joint
    B. Cartilaginous joint
    C. Gliding joint
    D. Fibrous joint.

15. A mallet finger injury affects the:
    A. Distal phalanx
    B. Digital nerve
    C. Interphalangeal joint
    D. Flexor digitorum longus.

16. In which one of the following conditions may sequestra occur?
    A. Osteoarthritis
    B. Acute osteomyelitis
    C. Chronic osteomyelitis
    D. Osteochondritis.

17. Which one of the following structures may be constricted in carpal tunnel syndrome?
    A. Median nerve
    B. Radial artery
    C. Ulnar nerve
    D. Ulnar artery.

18. Which one of the following may displace the distal fragment in a fracture of the lower third of the femur?
    A. Soleus muscle
    B. Quadriceps muscle
    C. Patella tendon
    D. Gastrocnemius muscle.

19. Passive movement of the right leg would be unsuitable for which one of the following?
    A. An unconscious patient
    B. A patient with a fractured shaft of right femur
    C. A patient with a right hemiplegia
    D. A paraplegic patient.

20. A Baker's cyst is a:
    A. Fatty cyst over the patella
    B. Dermoid cyst of the palm seen in bakers
    C. Synovial cyst in the popliteal fossa
    D. Ganglion on the dorsum of the wrist.

21. The commonest site of acute osteomyelitis in the growing bone is the:
    A. Epiphysis
    B. Diaphysis
    C. Symphysis
    D. Metaphysis.

22. Reactionary haemorrhage occurs:
    A. At the time of the operation
    B. Ten days after the operation
    C. When the blood pressure returns to normal
    D. As a result of an infection.

23. How many pairs of chromosomes are there in the human cell?
    A. 22
    B. 23
    C. 24
    D. 25.

24. Trisomic No. 21 chromosomes are found in:
    A. Down's syndrome
    B. Muscular dystrophy
    C. Turner's syndrome
    D. Osteogenesis imperfecta.

25. Plantar flexion of the ankle joint, inversion of the sub-talar joint and adduction of the mid-tarsal joints are the deformities found in:
    A. Talipes calcaneo-valgus
    B. Talipes equino-varus
    C. Vertical talus
    D. Pes cavus.

26. Which of the following is the correct action if a patient develops respiratory difficulty and cyanosis when recovering from an anaesthetic?
    A. Check the pulse and blood pressure
    B. Start external cardiac massage
    C. Attempt to clear the airway
    D. Summon the 'cardiac arrest team'.

27. Three days after a blow to the upper end of the tibia, a 7-year-old boy becomes acutely ill and complains of pain over the area. He is most likely suffering from:
    A. Acute rheumatism
    B. Tuberculosis
    C. Acute osteomyelitis
    D. Osgood-Schlatter disease.

28. Which of the following drugs is not usually used in the treatment of tuberculosis?
    A. Sulphathiazole
    B. Isoniazid
    C. Ethambutol
    D. Rifampicin.

29. Which of the following is the most common treatment for a new born baby who has congenital talipes equino-varus?
    A. The feet will be observed until the child is 1 year old and then treatment will commence
    B. Surgical correction will be carried out as soon as possible
    C. Plaster of Paris will be applied after correcting the deformity
    D. The feet will be manipulated and held in the corrected position by strapping.

30. The commonest infecting organism in osteomyelitis is:
    A. *Staphylococcus aureus*
    B. *Streptococcus faecalis*
    C. *Clostridium welchii*
    D. *Pseudomonas aeruginosa*.

31. Which of the following terms does *not* apply to the pathological changes taking place in osteomyelitis?
    A. Involucrum
    B. Sequestrum
    C. Bulla
    D. Cloaca.

32. A Velpeau bandage may be used:
    A. As a substitute for plaster of Paris
    B. To immobilize the arm in fractures of the humerus
    C. To control swelling of the knee after injury
    D. To maintain the corrected position of a club foot after manipulation.

33. Following a supracondylar fracture of the humerus Volkmann's ischaemic contracture may occur due to damage to the:
    A. Radial nerve
    B. Median nerve
    C. Ulnar artery
    D. Brachial artery.

34. Which one of the following statements does *not* apply to Paget's disease?
    A. The circumference of the head may increase
    B. Bowing of the legs occurs
    C. It can lead to sarcoma of the bone
    D. It is commoner in women than men.

35. Which of the following drugs would be used in the treatment of gout?
    A. Allopurinol
    B. Ibuprofen
    C. Prednisolone
    D. Calcitonin.

36. A March fracture is a:
    A. Fracture-dislocation of the thumb
    B. Fatigue fracture of the metatarsals
    C. Fracture-dislocation of the ankle
    D. Pathological fracture in Paget's disease.

37. Which of the following statements does *not* apply to a lesion of the axillary (circumflex) nerve?
    A. It may be damaged in a dislocation of the shoulder
    B. The arm cannot be abducted
    C. The treatment consists of bandaging the arm to the side.
    D. There is a small area of anaesthesia over the lower part of the deltoid.

38. Neuropraxia means:
    A. Complete division of a nerve and its surrounding sheath
    B. Compression of the axon without rupture of the sheath
    C. Temporary damage to the sheath with the axon still intact
    D. Damage to the sensory nerve only.

39. Which one of the following is *not* usually associated with ankylosing spondylitis?
    A. The presence of a HLA B27 antigen
    B. A positive 'rheumatoid factor'
    C. Ligamentous calcification giving a 'bamboo spine' appearance on X-ray
    D. Ankylosis of the sacro-iliac joints.

40. Which one of the following drugs may be injected into a joint to produce a 'medical synovectomy' in rheumatoid arthritis?
    A. Hydrocortisone acetate
    B. Dexamethasone
    C. Radioactive yttrium 90
    D. Mefenamic acid.

41. When giving steroid treatment to a patient with rheumatoid arthritis, which of the following would most probably be prescribed as a maintenance dose?
    A. Hydrocortisone 15 mg three times a day
    B. Betamethasone 5 mg daily
    C. Corticotrophin 80 units daily
    D. Prednisolone 2 mg twice a day.

42 Which one of the following is *not* generally considered to be a side-effect of steroid therapy?
    A. Paranoia
    B. Osteoporosis
    C. Thrombocytopenia
    D. Sodium retention.

True/false statements *(Answers to Q. 1–100 appear on p. 147)*
The questions in this section are made up of statements which may be true or false. Study each statement and decide whether you consider it to be true or false.

1–4. In the spine:
1. The sacral curve is a primary curve
2. The cervical curve is present at birth
3. The lumbar curve develops when the baby sits and walks
4. The thoracic curve is concave forward.

5–8. The femur:
5. Has an angle of 100° between the neck and the shaft
6. Bows forwards and slightly inwards
7. Has a posterior roughened surface for the attachment of the interosseous membrane
8. Has the insertion of gluteus medius and minimus at the greater trochanter.

9–12. One of the following nerves supplies both the hip and the knee:
9. Obturator
10. Femoral
11. Sciatic
12. Peroneal.

13–16. The dura mater:
13. Is attached to the edge of the foramen magnum
14. Forms a covering for the spinal nerve roots as they form the spinal nerves
15. Lines the inner surface of the skull
16. Extends downwards in the vertebral canal no further than the first sacral nerve.

17–20. The pia mater:
17. Is avascular
18. Is tough and fibrous
19. Follows the convolutions of the brain
20. Forms the filum terminale at the lower end of the cord.

21–24. The following ligaments give stability to the vertebral column:
21. Lateral ligament
22. Ligamentum teres
23. Anterior longitudinal ligament
24. Ligamentum flavum.

25–28. The shoulder joint:
25. Is the joint between the acromion process and the head of humerus
26. Is very stable
27. Has the long head of biceps extra-capsular
28. Is strengthened by the coraco-humeral ligament.

29–32. In the hand:
29. The interosseous muscles lie between the metacarpal bones
30. The ulnar nerve supplies the skin of the lateral surfaces
31. The interphalangeal joints are hinge-type joints
32. Contraction of the thenar muscles produces opposition of the thumb.

33–36. In the foot:
33. Inversion and eversion occur at the sub-talar joint
34. Muscles and ligaments support the bony arches
35. The short muscles are supplied by the common peroneal nerve
36. The intertarsal joints are hinge-type joints.

37–40. The following blood tests are diagnostic tests for rheumatoid athritis:
37. Widal
38. Rose-Waaler
39. Paul-Bunnell
40. Sheep cell agglutination test.

41–44. Trendelenburg's sign is positive:
41. When there is paralysis of the gluteal muscles
42. If the pelvis drops on the affected side when the patient stands on the affected leg
43. In an 18-month old child with untreated congenital dislocation of the hip
44. In a 6-year-old child with Perthes' disease.

45–48. Coxa vara deformity may result from:
- 45. Slipped upper femoral epiphysis
- 46. Osteoarthritis of the hip
- 47. Paget's disease
- 48. Malunion of a fractured neck of femur.

49–52. Spondylolisthesis:
- 49. Is the backward displacement of the vertebral body compressing the spinal cord
- 50. May be caused by a congenital defect in the development of the neural arch
- 51. Rarely occurs in people under the age of 50
- 52. Can cause root pain and sciatica.

53–56. Klumpke's paralysis:
- 53. Results from damage to the C5, C6 and C7 nerve roots
- 54. Is associated with a breech delivery
- 55. Affects the intrinsic muscles of the hand and finger flexors
- 56. Sometimes follows a traction injury to the arm, especially in motorcycle accidents.

57–60. Closed reduction of a congenital dislocation of the hip may not be achieved because:
- 57. There is hypertrophy of the ligamentum teres
- 58. The acetabular labrum is inverted
- 59. There is dysplasia of the acetabulum
- 60. The joint capsule is contracted.

61-64. In tetanus:
- 61. The organism flourishes in aerobic conditions
- 62. The organism produces an endotoxin which affects the brain
- 63. A child under 1 year has an inborn immunity to the disease
- 64. Tetanus toxoid gives an active immunity against the disease.

65–68. The following clinical features may be seen in advanced rheumatoid arthritis:
- 65. Ulnar deviation of the fingers
- 66. 'Dinner fork' deformity of the wrist
- 67. 'Swan neck' deformity of the fingers
- 68. Heberden's nodes.

69–72. In Erb's palsy:

69. There is damage to C5, C6 and C7 nerve roots
70. The arm is carried in the 'porter's tip' position
71. Treatment is to strap the arm to the side
72. Full recovery rarely occurs.

73–76. In spastic-type cerebral palsy:

73. The lesion is of the lower motor neuron
74. There is an inability to perform co-ordinated movements
75. Flexion, adduction and medial rotation of the affected hip is a common deformity
76. Tendon reflexes are decreased.

77–80. Damage to the radial nerve:

77. Leads to wrist drop
78. Can result from a dislocated shoulder
79. Causes anaesthesia of the palm of the hand and fingers
80. May be compressed in 'carpal tunnel syndrome'.

81–84. Slipped upper femoral epiphysis:

81. Frequently occurs in adolescent boys
82. Is usually due to a disturbance in the secretion of sex hormones
83. Is always treated surgically
84. Rarely affects both hips.

85–88. Pressure on the lateral popliteal (common peroneal) nerve from a long leg plaster of Paris would be indicated by:

85. Numbness or tingling of the toes
86. Blueness of the toes
87. Inability to extend the toes
88. Pressure over the head of fibula.

89–92. When drying a single plaster of Paris hip spica the nurse should:

89. Handle the cast with the palms of the hands
90. Support the cast on hard pillows covered with turkish towelling
91. Keep the patient in the recumbent position until the plaster is dry
92. Turn the patient with the unplastered leg uppermost.

93–96. When applying long leg extensions the nurse should make sure that:

93. The knee is covered by the bandage
94. The extension strapping does not cover the tibial crest
95. Small diagonal cuts are made at the edges of the strapping to allow moulding
96. Bandaging begins proximal to the malleoli

97–100. The following safety points should be followed on the children's ward;

97. Dummies should not be allowed
98. Restrainers should only be used if advised by the paediatrician
99. Hot water bottles can be used if covered
100. Steam kettles should only be used if prescribed.

Matching item questions *(Answers to Q. 1–90 appear on p. 48)*

The questions in this section are of the matching item type. They consist of two lists—the list on the left is of items lettered A, B, C etc, and the lists on the right consists of items numbered 1, 2, and 3. When you have studied the two lists choose the appropriate item from the lettered list on the left which corresponds to each one of the items in the right hand numbered list.

N.B. There are more items in the lettered list on the left than in the numbered list on the right so all the items in the lettered list will not be used.

1–3. From the list on the left select the appropriate definition of each word listed on the right.

A. Nearest to the axis of the body
B. Bring towards the axis of the body
C. Nearest to the head
D. In front
E. Behind

1. Proximal
2. Medial
3. Dorsal

4–6. From the list on the left select the type of joint which each joint listed on the right is an example.

A. Pivot
B. Saddle
C. Ball and socket
D. Ellipsoid
E. Hinge

4. Wrist
5. Atlanto-axial
6. Interphalangeal

7–9. From the list on the left select a movement which can be produced by each muscle listed on the right.

A. Rotates the arm medially
B. Abducts the arm
C. Rotates the arm laterally
D. Flexes the elbow
E. Extends the elbow.

7. Brachialis
8. Deltoid
9. Subscapularis.

10–12. From the list on the left select a movement which can be produced by each muscle listed on the right.

A. Adducts the arm
B. Rotates the arm laterally
C. Flexes the elbow
D. Pronates the forearm
E. Extends the elbow.

10. Triceps
11. Pectoralis major
12. Biceps

13–15. From the list on the left select a movement which can be produced by each muscle listed on the right.

A. Abducts the hip
B. Adducts the hip
C. Laterally rotates the femur
D. Flexes the hip
E. Extends the hip.

13. Ilio-psoas
14. Gluteus maximus
15. Gluteus medius.

16–18. From the list on the left select a movement which can be produced by each muscle listed on the right.

A. Extends the hip
B. Rotates the femur medially
C. Abducts the hip
D. Extends the knee
E. Adducts the hip

16. Biceps femoris
17. Quadriceps femoris
18. Sartorius.

19–21. From the list on the left select a movement which can be produced by each muscle listed on the right.

A. Dorsiflexes the foot
B. Everts the foot
C. Plantarflexes the foot
D. Extends the knee
E. Extends the great toe.

19. Gastrocnemius
20. Tibialis anterior
21. Peroneus.

22–24. From the list on the left select the nerve which supplies each of the muscles listed on the right.

A. Axillary (circumflex)
B. Median
C. Musculo-cutaneous
D. Ulnar
E. Radial.

22. Brachialis
23. Triceps
24. Deltoid.

25–27. From the list on the left select the nerve which supplies each of the muscles listed on the right.

A. Obturator
B. Tibial
C. Femoral
D. Common peroneal
E. Sciatic.

25. Tibialis anterior
26. Quadriceps femoris
27. Biceps femoris.

28–30. From the list on the left select the description which most closely describes each type of exercise listed on the right.

A. The patient moves the limb with help
B. The patient moves the limb freely without outside assistance or restraint
C. The patient contracts the muscles without moving the underlying joint
D. The patient exercises the limb against a force such as a weight.
E. The physiotherapist puts the limb through a full range of movements.

28. Free active exercises
29. Isometric exercises
30. Resisted active exercises.

31- 33. From the list on the left select the definition of each word listed on the right.

A. Tumour of a nerve
B. Primitive nerve cell
C. Excision of a nerve
D. Supporting tissue of the brain and cord
E. Degeneration of a nerve.

31. Neuroglia
32. Neuroma
33. Neurectomy.

34–36. From the list on the left select the condition which results from a deficiency of each vitamin listed on the right.

A. Scurvy
B. Impaired blood clotting
C. Beri-beri
D. Rickets
E. Pernicious anaemia.

34. Vitamin B_{12}
35. Vitamin D
36. Vitamin K.

37–39. From the list on the left select the appropriate definition for each of the terms listed on the right.

A. Increased angle between the neck and the shaft of the femur
B. Decreased angle between the neck and the shaft of the femur
C. Knock knees
D. Bow leg
E. Backward bowing of the knees.

37. Coxa vara
38. Genu valgum
39. Genu recurvatum.

40–42. From the list on the left select the tissues which are chiefly affected in each of the conditions listed on the right.

A. Synovial membrane
B. Periosteum
C. Hyaline cartilage
D. Myelin sheath
E. Meninges.

40. Osteoarthritis
41. Rheumatoid arthritis
42. Multiple sclerosis.

43–45. From the list on the left select the appropriate definition of each condition listed on the right.

A. Thickening of the digital sheath of the flexor tendon of the finger
B. Contracture of the palmar aponeurosis
C. Cystic swelling on the dorsum of the wrist
D. Fibrous constriction of the sheaths of the extensor and abductor tendons of the thumb
E. Osteochondritis of the carpal lunate

43. De Quervain's syndrome
44. Trigger finger
45. Dupuytren's contracture.

46–48. From the list on the left select the bone which, when affected by osteochondritis, results in each disease listed on the right.

A. Lunate
B. Vertebra
C. Head of femur
D. Tibial tuberosity
E. Navicular

46. Osgood-Schlatter disease
47. Kienboeck's disease
48. Scheuermann's disease.

49–51. From the list on the left select the test or sign which may be used to aid the diagnosis of each condition listed on the right.

A. Trendelenburg's sign
B. Straight leg raising test
C. McMurray's test
D. Barlow's sign
E. Heaf's test.

49. Prolapsed intervertebral disc
50. Tuberculosis
51. Congenital dislocation of the hip in a newborn baby

52–54. From the list on the left select the appropriate definition of each condition listed on the right.

A. Damage to the common extensor origin of the elbow
B. Osteochondritis of the tibial tuberosity
C. Prepatellar bursitis
D. Olecranon bursitis
E. Damage to the common flexor origin of the elbow.

52. Housemaid's knee
53. Tennis elbow
54. Golfer's elbow.

55–57. From the list on the left select the predisposing condition which may lead to each condition listed on the right.

A. Scheuermann's disease
B. Perthes' disease
C. Osteoporosis
D. Osteomalacia
E. Tonsillitis

55. Colles' fracture
56. Osteomyelitis
57. Early osteoarthritis of the hip.

58–60. From the list on the left select the appropriate splint which may be used when treating each condition listed on the right.

A. Milwaukee brace
B. Bell Grice splint
C. Frejka pillow
D. Jones posterior spinal support
E. Rizzoli splint.

58. Congenital talipes equino-varus
59. Scoliosis
60. Congenital dislocation of the hip.

61–63. From the list on the left select the nerve which may be involved in each injury listed on the right.

A. Ulnar
B. Axillary (circumflex)
C. Musculo-cutaneous
D. Radial
E. Median.

61. Fractured surgical neck of humerus
62. Fractured mid-shaft of humerus
63. Dislocation of the lunate

64–66. From the list on the left select the appropriate test or sign which may be used to assist the diagnosis of each condition listed on the right.

A. Thomas' test
B. Babinski's sign
C. Trendelenburg's sign
D. Mantoux test
E. McMurray's sign.

64. Torn meniscus
65. Flexion contracture of the hip
66. Untreated congenital dislocation of the hip in a child who is walking.

67–69. From the list on the left select the most probable complication which may occur with each condition listed on the right.

A. Sciatic scoliosis
B. Sarcoma
C. Erb's palsy
D. Tetraplegia
E. Hydrocephalus

67. Paget's disease
68. Myelo-meningocele
69. Prolapsed intervertebral disc.

70–72. From the list on the left select the type of traction which may be used in the treatment of each condition listed on the right.

A. Pugh's
B. Pelvic
C. Alvik
D. Halo-femoral
E. Bryant.

70. Congenital dislocation of the hip
71. Scoliosis
72. Fractured femur in the newborn.

73–75. From the list on the left select the appropriate condition for which each operation listed on the right may be performed.

A. Hallux valgus
B. Frozen shoulder
C. Pes cavus
D. Recurrent dislocation of the shoulder
E. Ingrowing toe nail.

73. Bankart's operation.
74. Zadek's operation
75. Keller's operation.

76–78. From the list on the left select the specific blood test which would be requested when diagnosing each of the conditions listed on the right.

A. Blood gases
B. Serum protein
C. Blood culture
D. Serum uric acid
E. Blood glucose.

76. Osteomyelitis
77. Gout
78. Gangrene

79–81. From the list on the left select the drug which may be used to treat each condition listed on the right.

A. Calcitonin
B. Sodium aurothiomalate
C. Ethambutol
D. Levadopa
E. Trimethoprim

79. Rheumatoid arthritis
80. Tuberculosis
81. Paget's disease.

82–84. From the list on the left select the condition for which each splint listed on the right would be used.

A. Axillary nerve palsy
B. Common peroneal nerve palsy
C. Radial nerve palsy
D. Valgus ankle deformity
E. Varus ankle deformity

82. Rizzoli splint
83. Littler Jones abduction splint
84. Outside iron, inside T-strap.

85–87. From the list on the left select the surgical procedure which may be performed for each condition listed on the right.

A. Low friction arthroplasty
B. Moore's prosthesis
C. Moore's pins
D. Acetabuloplasty
E. Girdlestone's procedure.

85. Slipped upper femoral epiphysis
86. Congenital dislocation of the hip
87. Subcapital fracture of the femur.

88–90. From the list on the left select the test which may be used to assist the diagnosis of each condition listed on the right.

A. Sheep cell agglutination test
B. HLA B27 antigen
C. Alphafetoprotein
D. Bence-Jones protein
E. Paul-Bunnel.

88. Ankylosing spondylitis
89. Rheumatoid arthritis
90. Multiple myeloma.

Matching item questions using diagrams *(Answers to Q. 1–147 appear on pp. 48–49)*
The questions in this section consist of a diagram with numbered parts. With each diagram there is a list of named structures (A, B, C etc.) Study the diagram and for each numbered part select the appropriate name from the list.

1–3 A section through a growing bone
- A. Medullary canal
- B. Epiphysis
- C. Diaphysis
- D. Epiphyseal cartilage
- E. Articular cartilage.

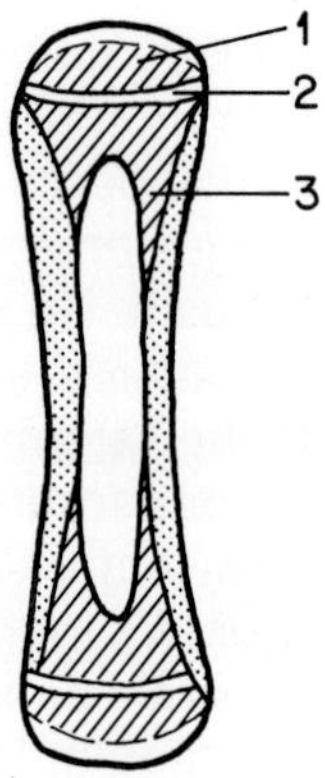

4–9 Longitudinal section through a long bone
- A. Periosteum
- B. Compact bone
- C. Medullary canal
- D. Articular cartilage
- E. Cancellous bone
- F. Red bone marrow
- G. Synovial membrane
- H. Epiphyseal line.

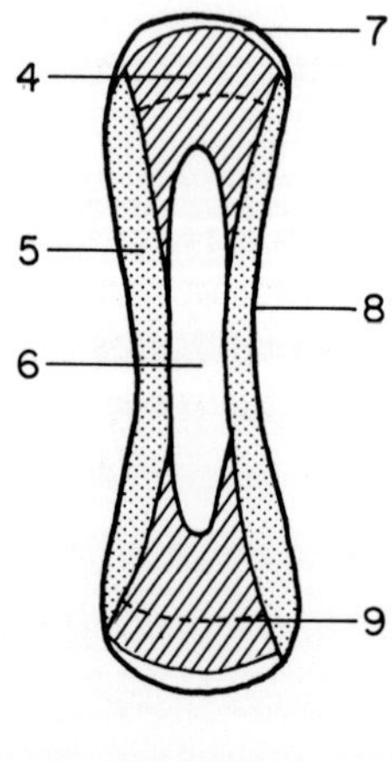

10–12 A section through a flat bone

A. Articular cartilage
B. Compact bone
C. Periosteum
D. Cancellous bone
E. Synovial membrane.

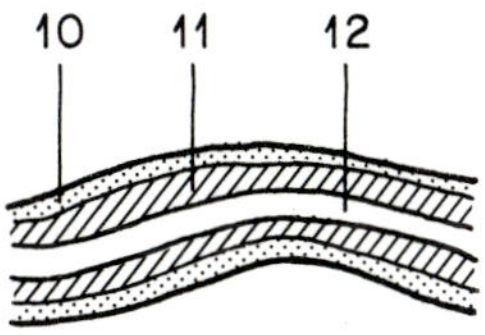

13–15 A section through a typical synovial joint

A. Articular cartilage
B. Periosteum
C. Fibrous capsule
D. Synovial membrane
E. Synovial fluid

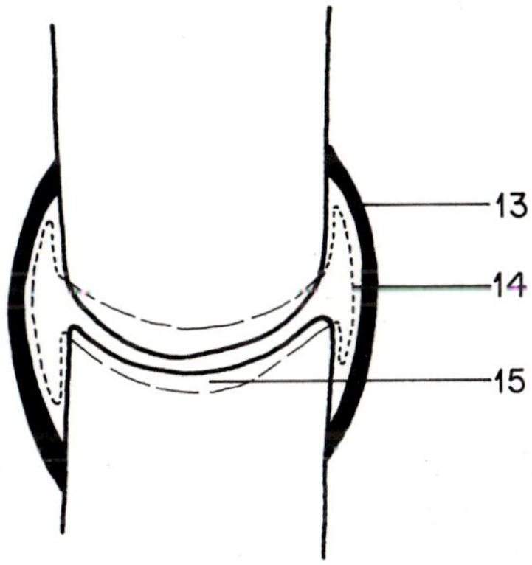

16–18 The atlas vertebra — superior view

A. Transverse process
B. Foramen for vertebral artery
C. Facet for odontoid process
D. Facet for occipital condyle
E. Anterior tubercle

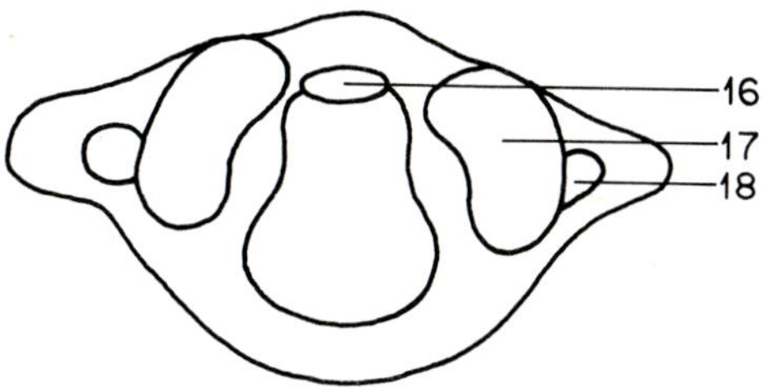

19–21 The axis vertebra — superior view
A. Facet for transverse ligament
B. Body
C. Facet for atlas
D. Odontoid process
E. Spinous process.

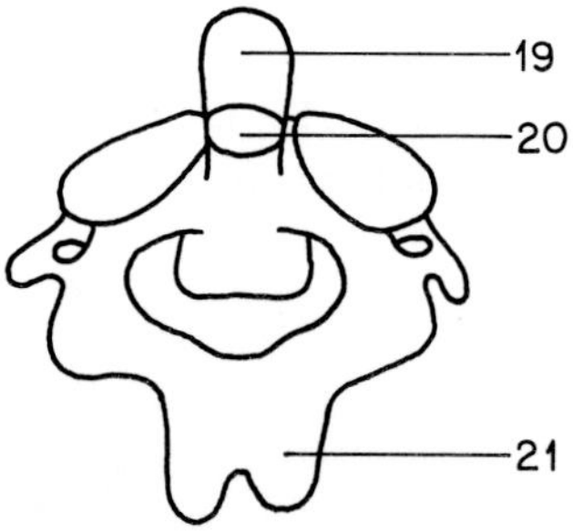

22–24 A typical cervical vertebra — superior view
A. Spinous process
B. Pedicle
C. Transverse process
D. Lamina
E. Vertebral foramen.

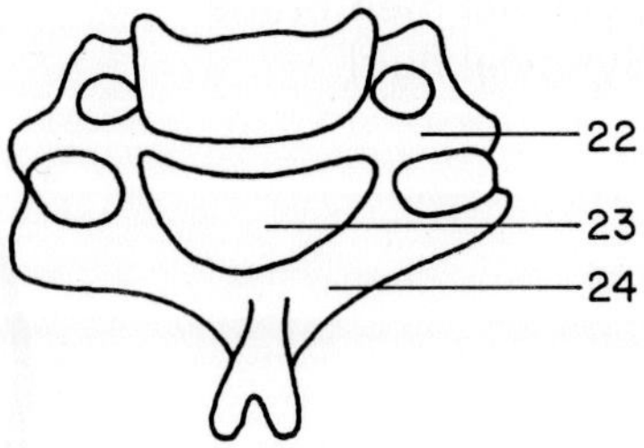

25–27 A typical thoracic vertebra — lateral view
A. Demi-facet of head of rib
B. Inferior articular process
C. Superior articular process
D. Articular surface for tubercle of the rib
E. Intervertebral notch.

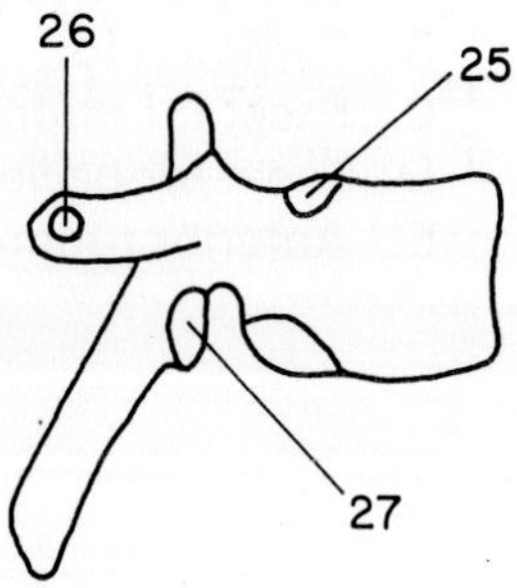

28–30 A typical lumbar vertebra—superior view

A. Spinous process
B. Lamina
C. Transverse process
D. Pedicle
E. Body.

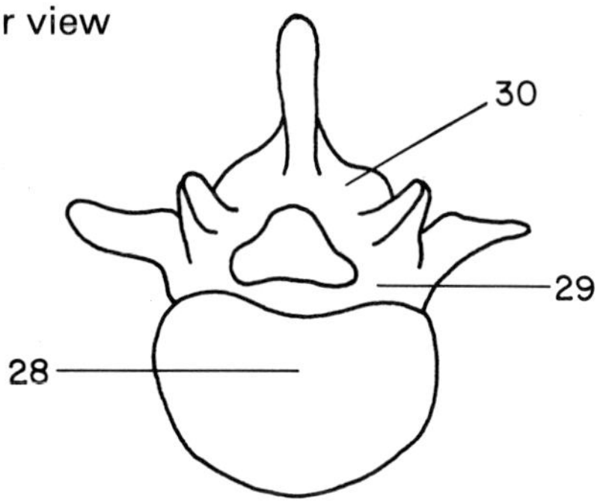

31–33 The sacrum and coccyx

A. Articulating surface for 5th lumbar vertebra
B. Superior articulating process
C. Coccyx
D. Foramen for sacral nerve
E. Surface for articulating with the ilium.

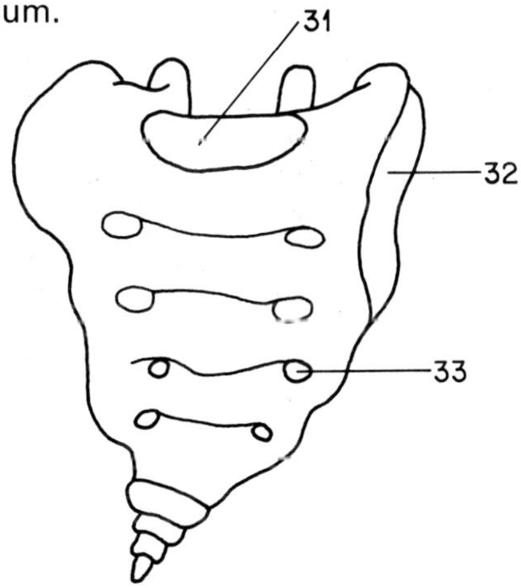

34–36 The sternum

A. Xiphoid process
B. Clavicular notch
C. Sternal angle
D. Suprasternal notch
E. Manubrium.

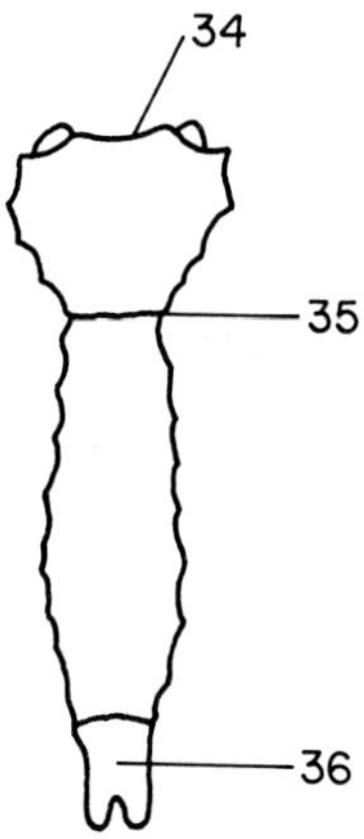

37–39 A typical rib
A. Shaft
B. Neck
C. Costal cartilage
D. Tubercle
E. Head

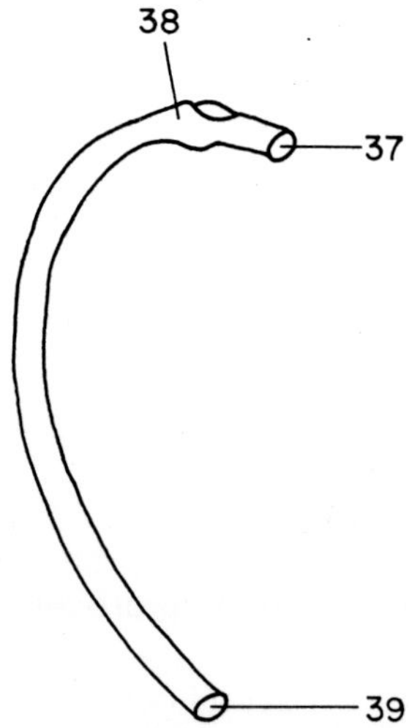

40–42 The right scapula—posterior view
A. Glenoid cavity
B. Coracoid process
C. Suprasternal fossa
D. Acromion process
E. Superior angle

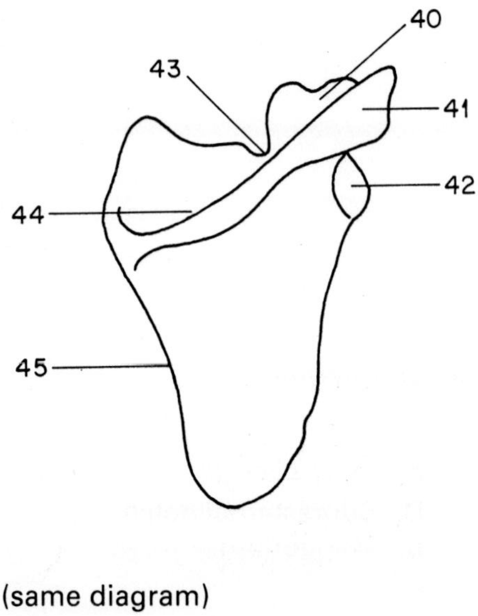

43–45 Posterior view of right scapula (same diagram)
A. Medial border
B. Infraspinous fossa
C. Supraspinous fossa
D. Lateral border
E. Suprascapular notch

46–48 The left humerus — anterior view
A. Anatomical neck
B. Surgical neck
C. Lesser tuberosity
D. Greater tuberosity
E. Bicipital groove.

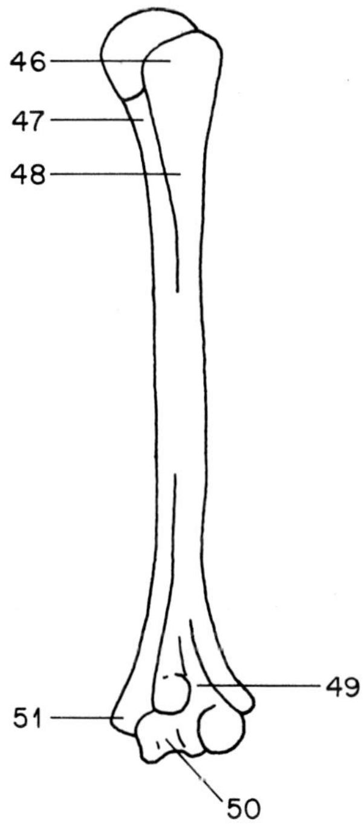

49–51 Anterior view of left humerus (same diagram)
A. Medial epicondyle
B. Olecranon fossa
C. Capitulum
D. Trochlea
E. Radial notch.

52–54 The left radius and ulna — anterior view

A. Ulnar tuberosity
B. Radial notch
C. Head of ulna
D. Olecranon process
E. Coronoid process

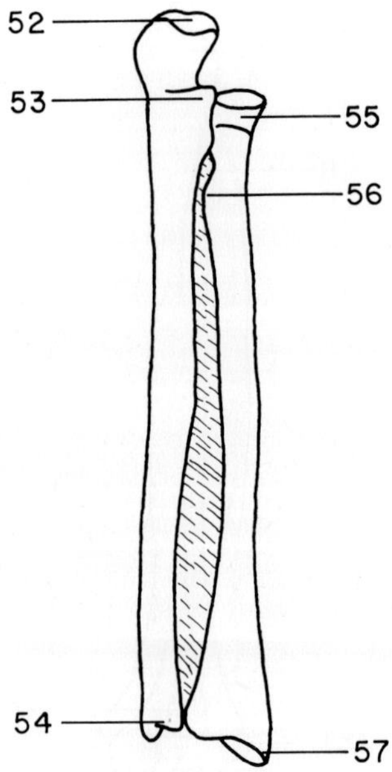

55–57 Anterior view of left radius and ulna (same diagram)

A. Interosseous membrane
B. Head of radius
C. Radial tuberosity
D. Shaft of radius
E. Styloid process

58–60 The bones of the wrist, hand and fingers
A. Proximal phalanx
B. Scaphoid
C. Distal phalanx
D. Lunate
E. Trapezium.

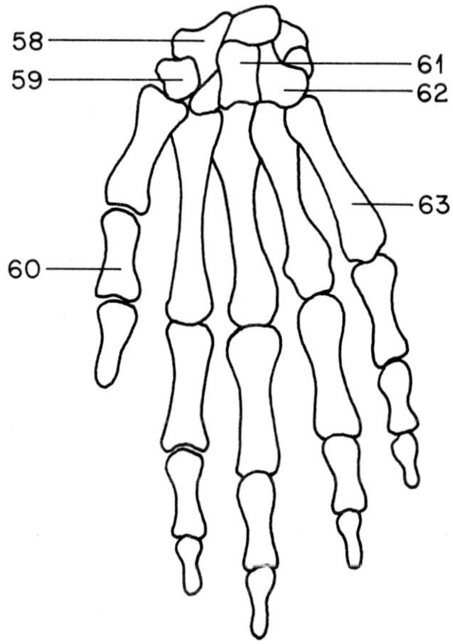

61–63 Right hand and wrist (same diagram)
A. 5th metacarpal
B. 1st metacarpal
C. Capitate
D. Trapezoid
E. Hamate

64–66 The right innominate bone — lateral view
- A. Greater sciatic notch
- B. Obturator foramen
- C. Lesser sciatic notch
- D. Acetabulum
- E. Anterior superior iliac spine.

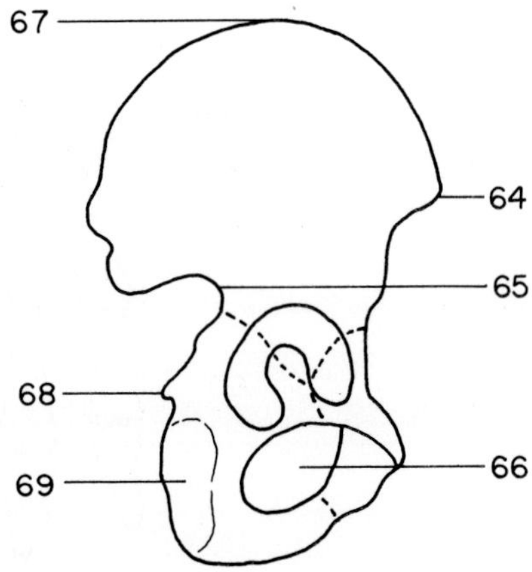

67–69 Lateral view of the right innominate bone (same diagram)
- A. Posterior superior iliac spine
- B. Ischial spine
- C. Iliac crest
- D. Symphysis pubis
- E. Ischial tuberosity.

70–72 The pelvis
- A. Ileopectineal line
- B. Iliac crest
- C. Sacro-iliac joint
- D. Ischial spine
- E. Pubis

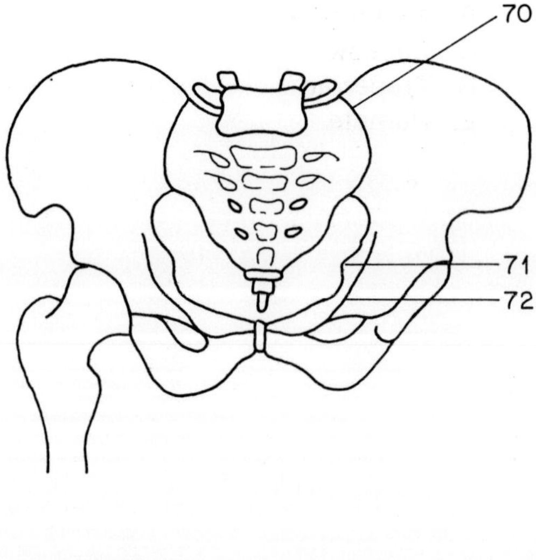

73–75 The left femur—posterior view
- A. Adductor tubercle
- B. Intertrochanteric line
- C. Greater trochanter
- D. Trochanteric fossa
- E. Linea aspera.

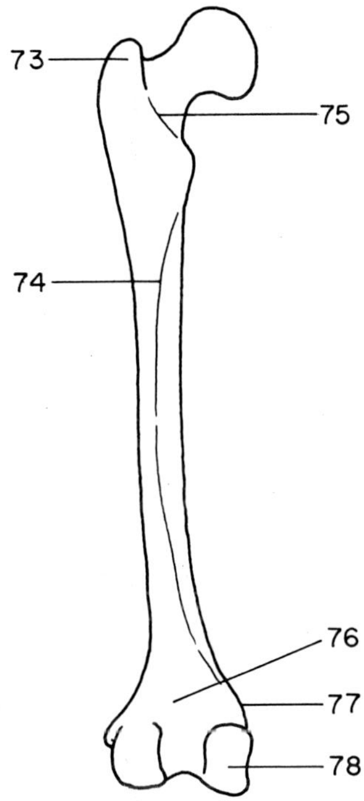

76–78 Posterior view of left femur (same diagram)
- A. Medial condyle
- B. Lesser trochanter
- C. Adductor tubercle
- D. Popliteal surface
- E. Intercondylar notch.

79–81 The right tibia and fibula — anterior view

A. Neck of fibula
B. Interosseous membrane
C. Lateral malleolus
D. Lateral condyle
E. Head of fibula.

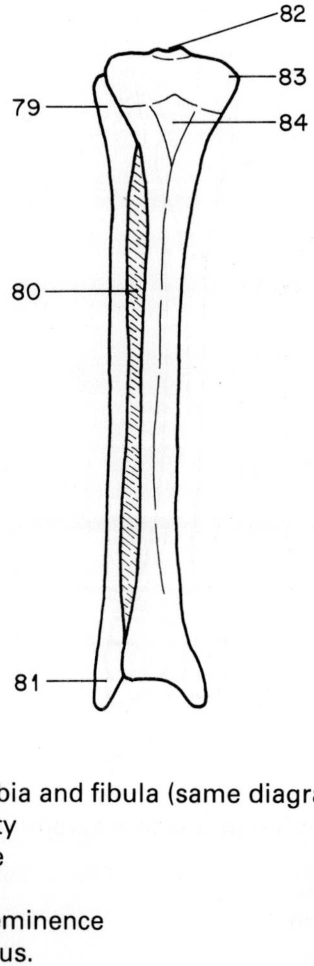

82–84 Anterior view of tibia and fibula (same diagram)

A. Tibial tuberosity
B. Medial condyle
C. Tibial crest
D. Intercondylar eminence
E. Medial malleolus.

85–87 The bones of the right foot—dorsal view
A. Talus
B. Cuneiform
C. Calcaneus
D. Cuboid
E. Navicular.

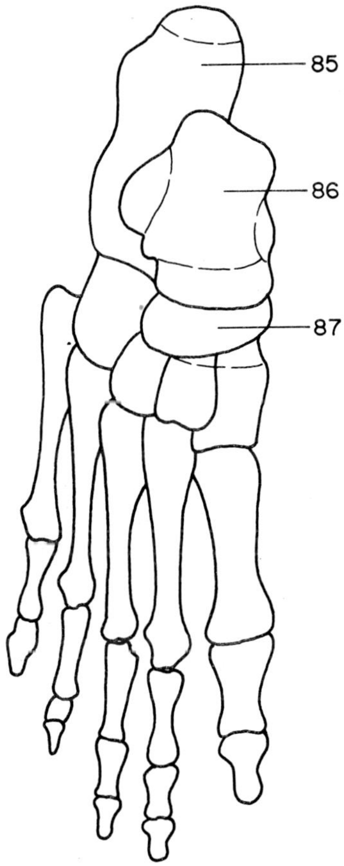

88–90 The shoulder joint — vertical section

A. Synovial cavity
B. Joint capsule
C. Synovial membrane
D. Long head of biceps muscle
E. Glenoid labrum.

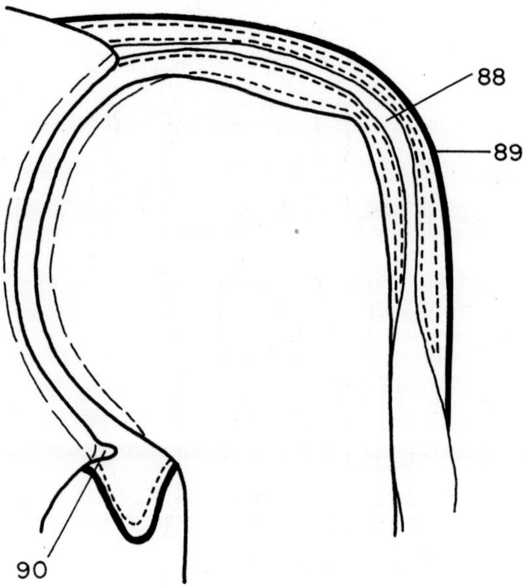

91–93 The right shoulder joint—anterior view

A. Coraco-acromial ligament
B. Transverse humeral ligament
C. Coracohumeral ligament
D. Middle glenohumeral ligament
E. Coracoclavicular ligament.

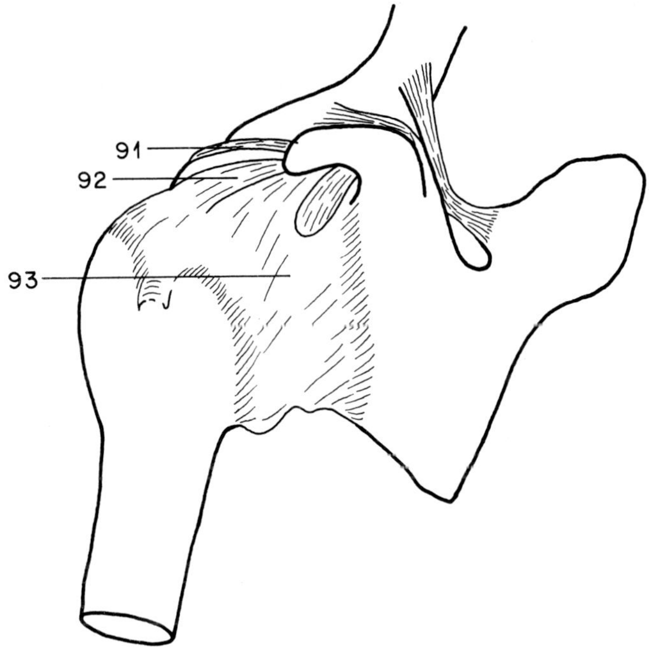

94–96 A section through the left elbow joint
A. Capsular ligament
B. Annular ligament
C. Coronoid process
D. Trochlear
E. Olecranon fossa.

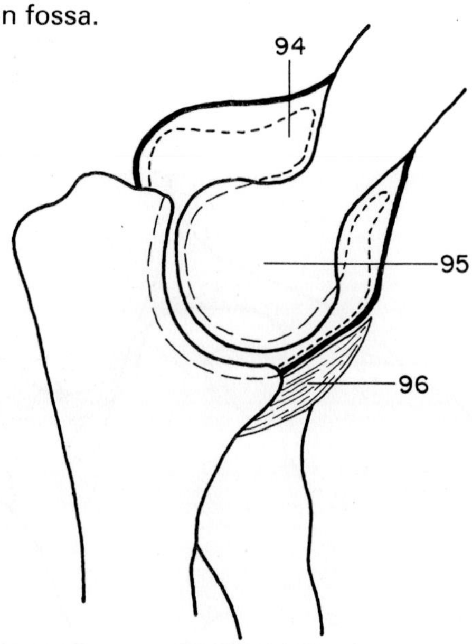

97–99 A section through the right wrist joint
A. Scaphoid
B. Ulnar collateral ligament
C. Cartilaginous disc
D. Triquetral
E. Inferior radio-ulnar joint.

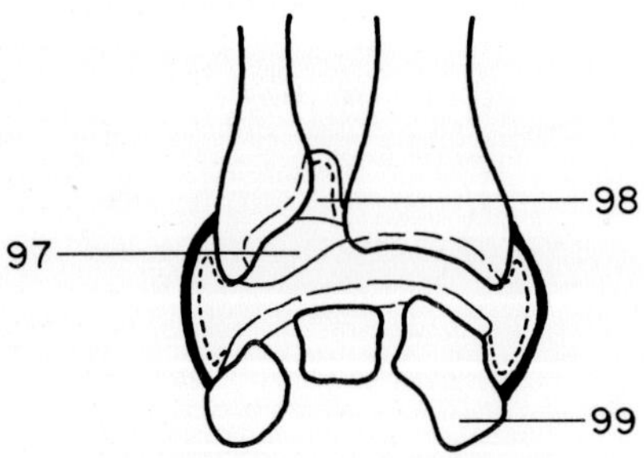

100–102 The hip joint—vertical section

A. Transverse ligament of acetabulum
B. Joint capsule
C. Pad of fat
D. Ligamentum teres
E. Acetabular labrum.

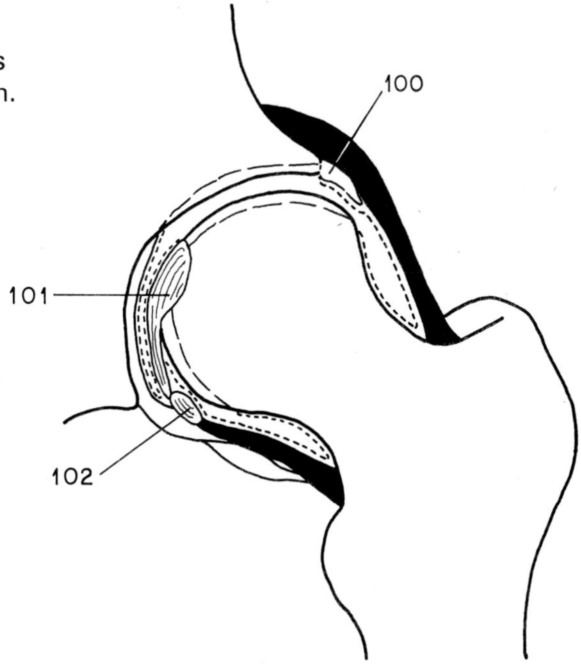

103–105 The right hip joint—anterior view

A. Iliopectineal line
B. Iliofemoral ligament
C. Trochanteric line
D. Ischiofemoral ligament
E. Pubofemoral ligament.

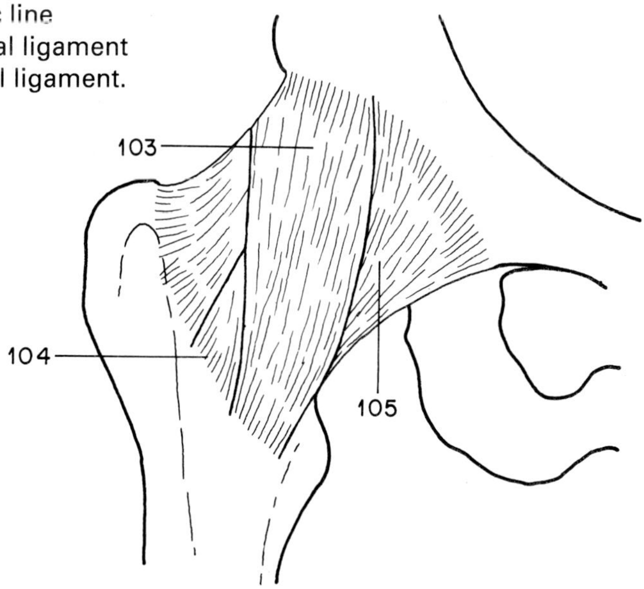

106–108 A coronal section through the knee joint

A. Synovial membrane
B. Fibrous capsule
C. Lateral meniscus
D. Medial meniscus
E. Cruciate ligament.

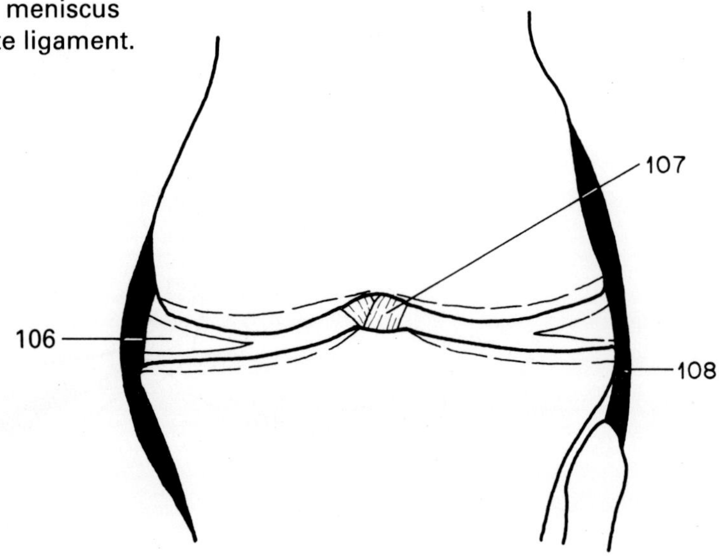

109–111 A coronal section through the ankle and subtalar joints

A. Deltoid ligament
B. Talocalcanean ligament
C. Posterior talofibular ligament
D. Talonavicular ligament
E. Anterior talofibular ligament.

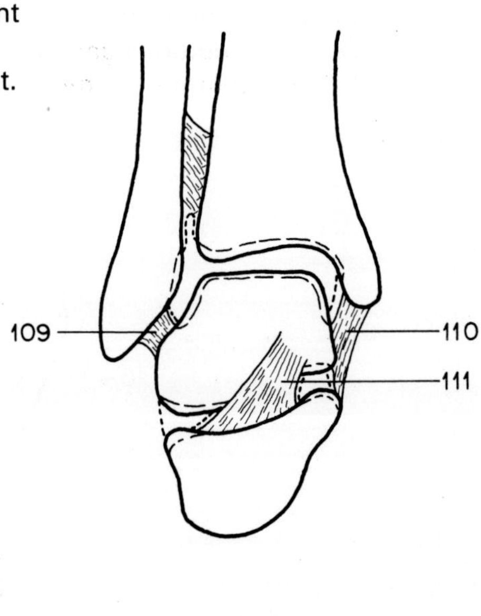

112–114 The muscles of the shoulder region — posterior view
A. Rhomboideus major
B. Lavator scapulae
C. Latissimus dorsi
D. Trapezius
E. Deltoid

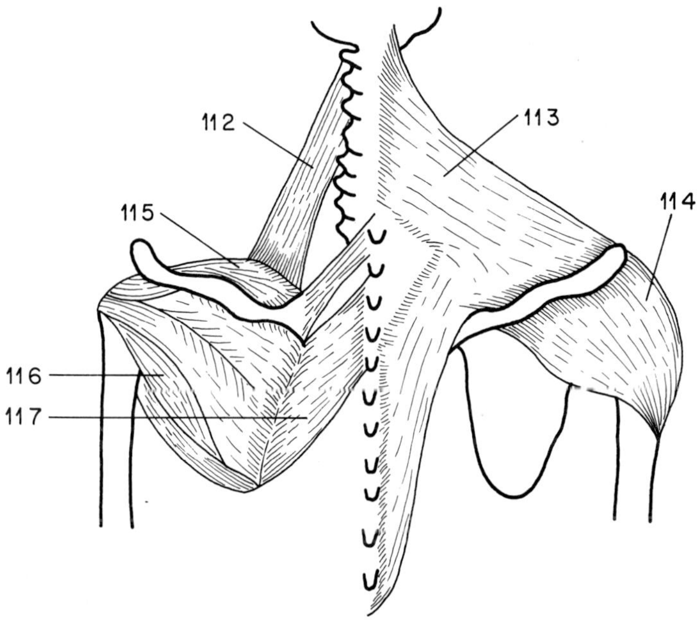

115–117 Posterior view of the muscles of the shoulder region (same diagram)
A. Supraspinatus
B. Teres major
C. Teres minor
D. Rhomboideus major
E. Infraspinatus.

118–120 The muscles of the upper arm — lateral view

A. Brachialis
B. Tendon of triceps
C. Long head of triceps
D. Short head of triceps
E. Long head of biceps

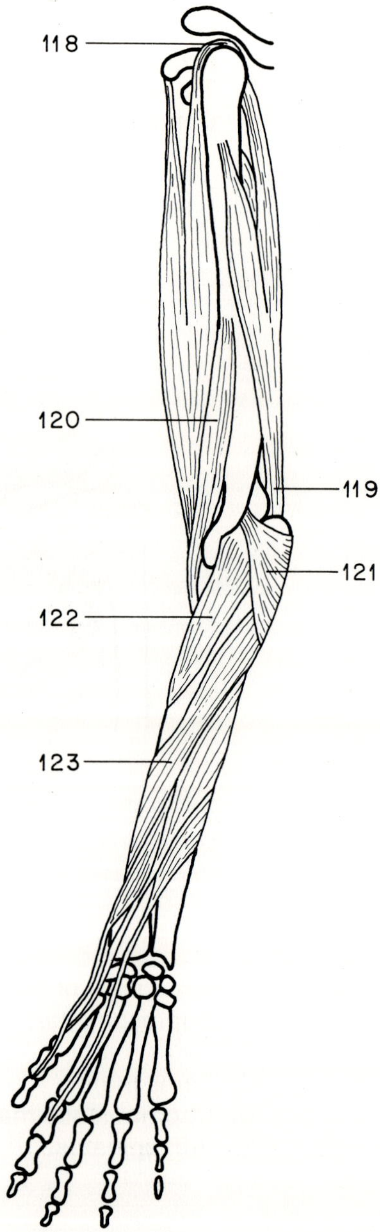

121–123 Lateral view of the forearm showing the deep muscles

A. Brachioradialis
B. Anconeus
C. Abductor pollicis longus
D. Supinator
E. Pronator teres.

124–126 The muscles forming the posterior abdominal wall

A. Sartorius
B. Psoas
C. Quadratus lumborum
D. Iliacus
E. Rectus femoris.

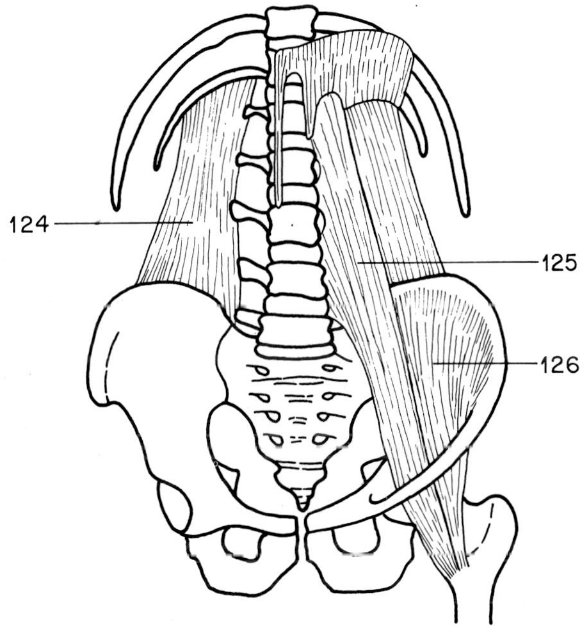

127–129 The muscles of the right thigh — anterior view

A. Sartorius
B. Rectus femoris
C. Vastus lateralis
D. Iliacus
E. Vastus medialis.

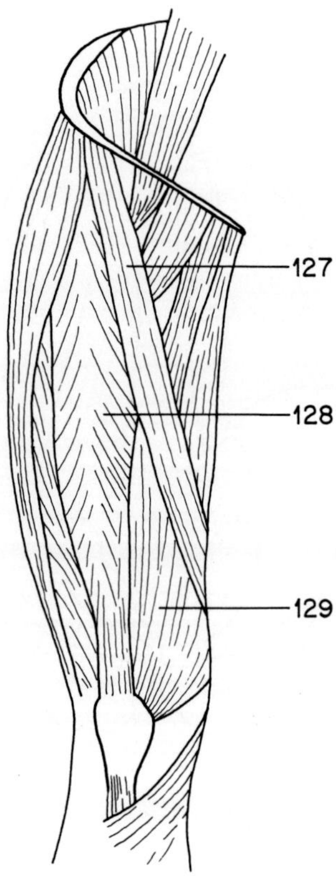

130–132 The muscles of the right thigh — posterior view
- A. Semitendinosus
- B. Semimembranosus
- C. Biceps femoris
- D. Gluteus maximus
- E. Gluteus medius.

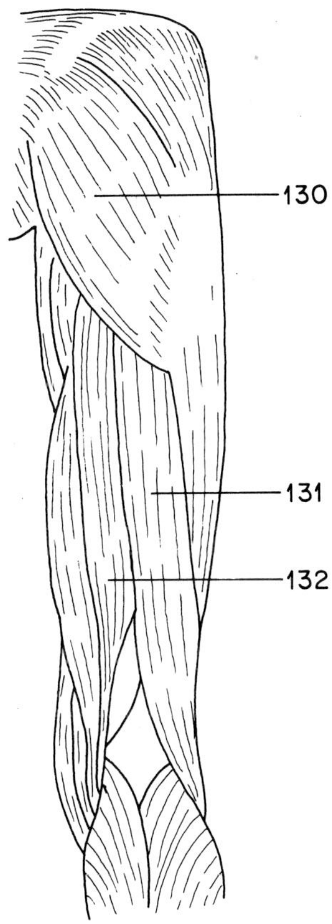

133–135 The muscles of the lower leg — anterior view

A. Soleus
B. Sartorius
C. Tibialis posterior
D. Tibialis anterior
E. Peroneus longus.

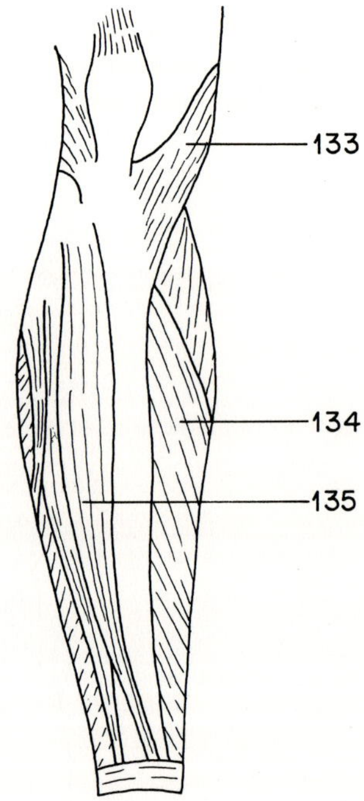

136–138 Diagram of the cervical and brachial plexes

A. Median nerve
B. Radial nerve
C. Phrenic nerve
D. Ulnar nerve
E. Musculo-cutaneous nerve.

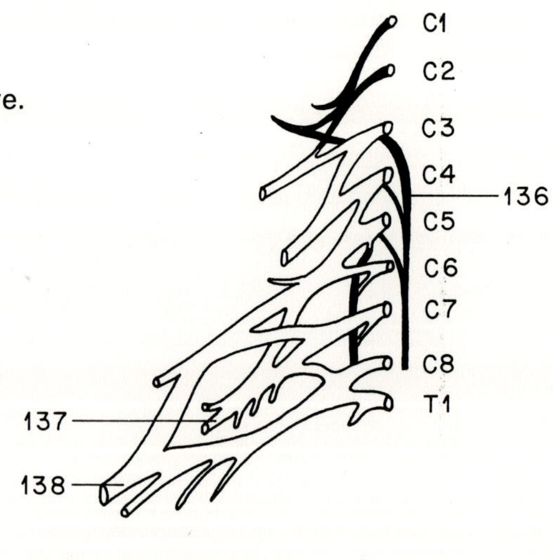

139–141 Diagram of the lumbar and sacral plexes

A. Femoral nerve
B. Obturator nerve
C. Great sciatic nerve
D. Pudendal nerve
E. Lateral cutaneous nerve.

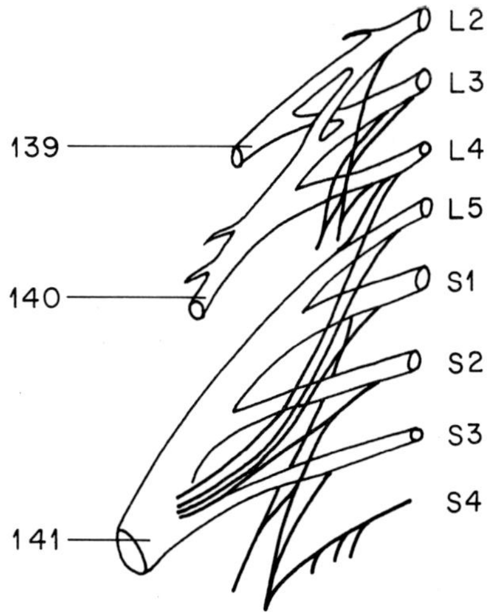

142–144 Diagram of the nerve supply to the arm — anterior view

A. Median nerve
B. Radial nerve
C. Musculo-cutaneous nerve
D. Ulnar nerve
E. Axillary nerve.

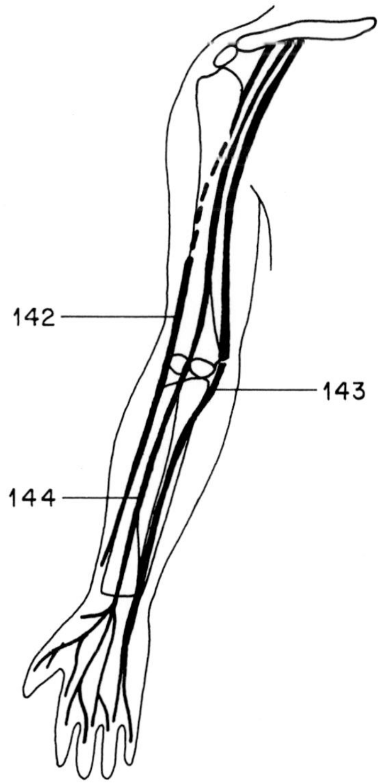

145–147 Diagram of the nerve supply to the leg — posterior view

A. Posterior tibial nerve
B. Sural nerve
C. Posterior cutaneous nerve
D. Pudendal nerve
E. Common peroneal nerve.

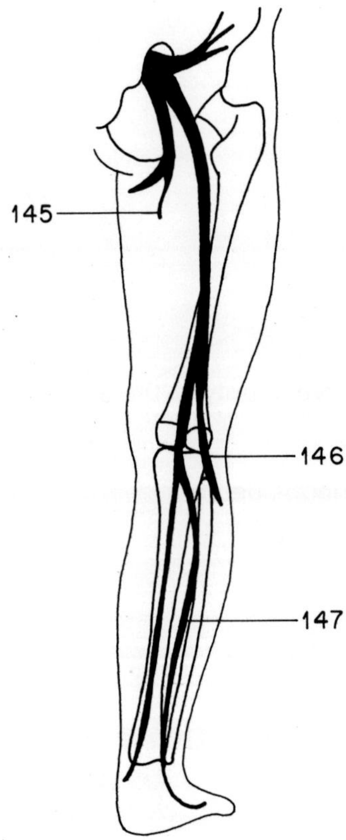

Answers to anatomy and physiology; orthopaedic conditions and trauma; orthopaedic nursing

Multiple choice questions

1. B	12. C	22. C.	32. B
2. A	13. D	23. B	33. D
3. A	14. B	24. A	34. D
4. B	15. A	25. B	35. A
5. D	16. C	26. C	36. B
6. C	17. A	27. C	37. C
7. D	18. D	28. A	38. C
8. A	19. B	29. D	39. B
9. C	20. C	30. A	40. C
10. B	21. D	31. C	41. D
11. C			42. C

True/false statements

1. True	26. False	51. False	76. False
2. False	27. False	52. True	77. True
3. True	28. True	53. False	78. False
4. True	29. True	54. True	79. False
5. False	30. False	55. True	80. False
6. True	31. True	56. False	81. True
7. False	32. True	57. True	82. True
8. True	33. True	58. True	83. False
9. True	34. True	59. True	84. False
10. True	35. False	60. False	85. True
11. False	36. False	61. False	86. False
12. False	37. False	62. False	87. True
13. True	38. True	63. False	88. True
14. True	39. False	64. True	89. True
15. True	40. True	65. True	90. True
16. False	41. True	66. False	91. False
17. False	42. False	67. True	92. False
18. False	43. True	68. False	93. False
19. True	44. False	69. True	94. True
20. True	45. True	70. True	95. True
21. False	46. False	71. False	96. False
22. False	47. True	72. False	97. False
23. True	48. True	73. False	98. True
24. True	49. False	74. True	99. False
25. False	50. True	75. True	100. True

Matching item questions

1. C
2. A
3. E
4. D
5. A
6. E
7. D
8. B
9. A
10. E
11. A
12. C
13. D
14. E
15. A
16. A
17. D
18. C
19. C
20. A
21. B
22. C
23. E
24. A
25. D
26. C
27. E
28. B
29. C
30. D
31. D
32. A
33. C
34. E
35. D
36. B
37. B
38. C
39. E
40. C
41. A
42. D
43. D
44. A
45. B
46. D
47. A
48. B
49. B
50. E
51. D
52. C
53. A
54. E
55. C
56. E
57. B
58. B
59. A
60. C
61. B
62. D
63. E
64. E
65. A
66. C
67. B
68. E
69. A
70. C
71. D
72. E
73. D
74. E
75. A
76. C
77. D
78. E
79. B
80. C
81. A
82. B
83. A
84. D
85. C
86. D
87. B
88. B
89. A
90. D

Matching item questions using diagrams

1. B
2. D
3. C
4. E
5. B
6. C
7. D
8. A
9. H
10. C
11. B
12. D
13. C
14. D
15. A
16. C
17. D
18. B
19. D
20. A
21. E
22. B
23. E
24. D
25. A
26. D
27. B
28. E
29. D
30. B
31. A
32. E
33. D
34. D
35. C
36. A
37. E
38. D
39. C
40. B
41. D
42. A
43. E
44. C
45. A
46. C
47. B
48. E
49. E
50. D
51. A
52. D
53. E
54. C
55. B
56. C
57. E
58. B
59. E
60. A
61. C
62. E
63. A
64. E
65. A
66. B
67. C
68. B
69. E
70. C
71. D
72. A
73. C
74. E
75. B
76. D
77. C
78. A
79. E
80. B
81. C
82. D
83. B
84. A
85. C
86. A
87. E
88. D
89. B
90. E
91. A
92. C
93. D
94. E
95. D
96. B
97. C
98. E
99. A
100. E
101. D
102. A
103. B
104. C
105. E
106. D
107. E
108. B
109. C
110. A
111. B
112. B
113. D
114. E
115. A
116. C
117. D
118. E
119. B
120. A
121. B
122. D
123. C
124. C
125. B
126. D
127. A
128. B
129. E
130. D
131. C
132. A
133. B
134. A
135. D
136. C
137. B
138. A
139. E
140. A
141. C
142. B
143. D
144. A
145. C
146. E
147. B

Section Two

This section consists of case histories on common orthopaedic conditions with related objective-type questions. As has been previously stated, the questions were not designed as an examination of knowledge at the end of a course but were written as an aid to learning and to help the student with revision.

The questions cover anatomy and physiology as applied to the condition, the pathology, the treatment and the nursing care. Wherever possible I have tried to incorporate the principles of the nursing process into the nursing care.

The answer section I have written in full, giving the reasons why I have chosen a particular answer as correct. I am sure there will be occasions when students will not agree with the answer which I have given and I hope that any controversial answers will stimulate discussion and further study. There is a bibliography at the end of the book, divided up by chapter, which the student may find useful.

When writing a case history I have obviously only been able to follow one line of treatment. The treatment of some orthopaedic conditions varies considerably from centre to centre so the method of treatment which I have selected may not be familiar to the individual student, e.g. the type of splintage. Students should refer to other textbooks for more detail about alternative methods of treatment and care.

The questions found in these case histories are of three types:

1. *True/false statements* where the student has to write down whether the given statement is true of false.
2. *Multiple choice questions* where the student has to select one correct answer from the list A–D.
3. *Matching item questions* which consist of two lists, the one on the left lettered A, B, C, etc. and the one on the right numbered 1,2,3. The student should choose the appropriate item from the lettered list on the left which fits each item on the num-

bered list on the right. N.B. There are more items in the lettered list on the left than the numbered list, so all the items in the lettered list will not be used.

The student should complete the case history before referring to the answer section.

Prolapsed intervertebral disc

Jim Williams, a 45-year-old farmer, is admitted to the general orthopaedic ward following a back injury which he sustained two weeks previously while carrying sacks of animal feed into his granary. That day he was unable to carry on working because of his pain and the next day his wife drove him to the surgery to see his family doctor.

On examination the doctor found that Mr Williams had severe pain in the lumbar region with limitation of movement and muscle spasm. He complained that the pain was worse on coughing or moving, and it radiated down his right leg to his calf. The doctor made a provisional diagnosis of acute prolapsed intervertebral disc with right-sided sciatica.

True/false statements *(Answers to Q. 1–11 appear on pp. 64–65)*
The following questions (1–11) are true/false statements about the structure of the vertebral column and the effects of injury upon it.

1. The vertebrae articulate with one another by cartilaginous and synovial joints.
2. The intervertebral discs form part of the synovial joints of the vertebral column.
3. The discs constitute approximately half the length of the spine.
4. The shape of the discs contributes to the anterior convex curves of the cervical and lumbar regions.
5. The intervertebral discs consist of a central nucleus pulposus and an outer annulus fibrosus.
6. The discs are entirely avascular.
7. Up to the age of about 20 years the only discs which are likely to be damaged by injury are those of the cervical region.

8. In adults, degenerative changes in the disc commonly lead to rupture of the annulus fibrosus and anterior protrusion of the nucleus pulposus.

9. Rupture of the intervertebral disc always causes pressure on an adjacent nerve root.

10. Spondylosis is frequently present where chronic disc degeneration has occurred.

11. Chronic degeneration of the intervertebral discs will lead to osteoarthritis of the intervertebral joints.

Multiple choice questions *(Answers to Q. 12–15 appear on pp. 66–67)*
The following questions (12–15) are multiple choice questions.

---

12. Injury to the intervertebral discs is most common in the cervical and lumbar regions of the spine because:
    A. Most movement occurs here and the discs tend to be frailer in these regions
    B. There are fewer bony supporting structures and the supporting ligaments are weaker
    C. Most movement occurs here and there are fewer bony supporting structures
    D. The discs tend to be frailer in these regions and the supporting ligaments are weaker.

13. In the lumbar region damage to the intervertebral discs occurs most commonly between:
    A. L1 and L2 vertebrae
    B. L2 and L3 vertebrae
    C. L3 and L4 vertebrae
    D. L5 and S1 vertebrae

14. Damage to the lumbar intervertebral discs occurs most commonly when the spine is flexed. Which of the following structures supports the spine in this position?
    A. Ligamenta flava, supraspinous ligament and interspinous ligaments
    B. Supraspinous ligament, interspinous ligaments and anterior longitudinal ligament
    C. Posterior longitudinal ligament, anterior longitudinal ligament and ligamenta flava
    D. Ligamentum teres, posterior longitudinal ligament and interspinous ligaments.

From Mr Williams' description of the pain down his leg, the doctor was able to diagnose pressure on the sciatic nerve. He told Mr Williams to go home to bed and to remain there for one week except for visits to the bathroom for bowel evacuation. A firm board was placed under Mr Williams' mattress and the doctor arranged for the social services to supply a urinal. The following prescription was given: indomethacin (Indocid) 25 mg three times a day; pentazocine (Fortral) 50 mg 4 hourly when required.

15. The sciatic nerve:
    A. Is formed from branches of the L2, L3, L4, L5 and S1 nerve roots and passes through the gluteal region under the gluteus medius muscle
    B. Passes down the medial aspect of the thigh under the hamstring muscle and divides just above the popliteal fossa to form the saphenous and common peroneal nerves
    C. Is formed from branches of the L4, L5, S1, S2 and S3 nerve roots and supplies the hamstring muscle
    D. Passes down the lateral aspect of the thigh and supplies the quadriceps femoris muscle.

True/false statements *(Answers to Q. 16–25 appear on pp. 67–68)*
The following questions (16–25) are true/false statements.

---

16. If Mr Williams has a period of bed-rest the prolapsed intervertebral disc may slip back into place.

17. Mrs Williams was told to place a firm board under her husband's mattress to support the normal curves of the spine.

18. If Mrs Williams could get a bedpan it would be better for her husband to use this in bed rather than go to the bathroom for bowel evacuation.

19. Mr Williams could wash and shave while he is in the bathroom.

20. Indomethacin will act on the damaged disc and the nerve roots.

21. Indomethacin should be taken between meals.

22. Gastric bleeding may occur suddenly, without previous gastro-intestinal symptoms, in people taking indomethacin for a long period.

23. Patients frequently complain of headaches and dizziness when they begin taking indomethacin.

24. The doctor should tell Mr Williams to take pentazocine (Fortral) if the pain gets very severe.

25. Mr Williams should be told to avoid drinking alcohol while taking pentazocine.

One week later the doctor called on Mr Williams and found that there was little improvement in his pain. An urgent appointment was made for him to see the orthopaedic surgeon and an ambulance was arranged to transport him to the hospital. Mr and Mrs Williams were warned that he might be admitted.

A detailed examination by the surgeon showed that Mr Williams had severe limitation of lumbar movement in all directions, restricted straight leg raising on the right side and weakness of dorsiflexion of the right great toe. Skin sensation was normal but the right ankle jerk reacted slowly when tested. Anterior/posterior and lateral X-rays showed no abnormality.

Multiple choice questions *(Answers to Q. 26–29 appear on p. 68)*
The following questions (26–29) are multiple choice questions.

26. Mr Williams' limited lumbar movement was most probably caused by:
    A. The vertebrae being locked
    B. Muscle spasm around the damaged disc
    C. Fear of causing more pain
    D. Stiffness due to the period spent in bed.

27. Weakness of dorsiflexion of the great toe is caused by pressure on the sciatic nerve. Which branch of the sciatic nerve supplies the muscles which dorsiflex the foot?
    A. Obturator nerve
    B. Tibial nerve
    C. Common peroneal nerve
    D. Pudendal nerve.

28. When the surgeon attempted to lift Mr Williams' right leg with the knee straight, increased pain prevented full movement because of:
    A. Stiffness of the hip from lying in bed
    B. Muscle spasm in the back
    C. Anxiety causing tension
    D. Stretching of the nerve root over the prolapsed disc.

29. X-rays of the spine would not show the prolapsed intervertebral disc. Which one of the following conditions giving similar symptoms could *not* be excluded from the diagnosis by these X-rays?
    A. Spondylolisthesis
    B. Tumour of the nerve root
    C. Osteoarthritis of the spine
    D. Ankylosing spondylitis.

The surgeon decided that Mr Williams should be admitted to the ward for a period of pelvic traction and for further investigations. He was admitted to the male orthopaedic ward and Nurse Little was assigned to care for him.

After leaving him for a short while to settle into his new environment she explained fully what the treatment involved and placed him onto pelvic traction with 3 kg weight on each cord and two pillows under his head. The foot of the bed was not elevated until the next morning.

True/false statements *(Answers to Q. 30–34 appear on pp. 68–70)*
The following questions (30–34) are true/false statements.

30. When explaining the traction treatment to Mr Williams Nurse Little would tell him that he must lie flat on his back at all times.
31. Mr Williams should be told to move his legs about as much as possible.
32. A bed cradle placed over Mr Williams' legs would increase the efficiency of the traction
33. A mirror placed over Mr Williams' bed would help him settle on the traction.
34. The foot of the bed was not elevated the first night because the weights on the traction were sufficient to begin the treatment.

Multiple choice questions *(Answers to Q. 35–38 appear on pp. 70–71)*
The following questions (35–38) are multiple choice questions.

35. Which of the following actions should Nurse Little take when Mr Williams complained of increased pain from lying flat a few hours after he had commenced his traction.
    A. Give him two more pillows under his head and one under his thighs
    B. Elevate the foot of the bed and give him analgesia
    C. Place a thin pillow under his thighs and give him analgesia
    D. Elevate the foot of his bed and give him two more pillows under his head.

36. During his time on traction, which of the following nursing procedures would Mr Williams require?
    A. Feeding by either the nursing staff or his wife and an accurate recording of his fluid intake and output
    B. An accurate recording of his fluid intake and output and a daily bed-bath
    C. Removal of the pelvic belt for treatment of the underlying skin and feeding by the nursing staff or his family
    D. A daily bed-bath and removal of the pelvic belt for treatment of the underlying skin.

37. Which one of the following would be the most suitable action for Nurse Little to take when Mr Williams' complained a few days later that he tended to be rather constipated since he had been confined to bed?
    A. Add bran to his cereal daily and allow him to sit on a commode at the bedside
    B. Give him daily suppositories and sit him on a bedpan with the elevator removed
    C. Administer an enema every third day and allow him to go to the toilet
    D. Give him aperients each evening and encourage him to use a slipper bedpan while lying flat.

When the surgeon saw Mr Williams one week later there was not much improvement in his pain or his nerve root signs. It was decided that surgery was necessary to remove the part of the disc which was pressing on the nerve root. Before this could be undertaken a radiculogram was performed to confirm the diagnosis and to identify the level of the prolapsed disc.

---

38. Between which lumbar vertebrae is the needle usually inserted when performing a radiculogram
    A. 1st and 2nd
    B. 2nd and 3rd
    C. 3rd and 4th
    D. 4th and 5th.

Matching item questions *(Answers to Q. 39–44 appear on pp. 71–72)*
The following questions (39–44) are matching item type questions.

39–41. From the list on the left select the appropriate injection given for each radiological test listed on the right.

A. Injection of contrast agent into the nucleus pulposus
B. Injection of a water soluble contrast agent into the subarachnoid space
C. Injection of a water soluble contrast agent into the epidural space
D. Injection of an oily-based contrast agent into the subarachnoid space
E. Injection of sterile water into the annulus fibrosus.

39. Myelography
40. Radiculography
41. Discography.

42–44. From the list on the left select the appropriate aftercare for a patient following each of the radiological tests listed on the right.

A. Nurse the patient lying in the lateral position
B. Encourage him to resume normal activities
C. Nurse him in the recumbent position with one pillow for 24 hours
D. Nurse him in the recumbent position with the foot of the bed elevated
E. Nurse him sitting up for 6 to 8 hours.

42. Myelography
43. Radiculography
44. Discography.

Five days later Mr Williams went into the operating theatre for an exploratory partial laminectomy and excision of the protruding part of the L5/S1 disc which had been identified as the cause of his pain. The operation proceeded without complication and his recovery from the anaesthetic was uneventful. The post-operative instructions were that Mr Williams should be nursed in the recumbent position for the first 4 hours and then he should be turned from side to side 2 hourly.

Mr Williams had two vacuum drainage tubes from his wound, and an intravenous infusion of Normal saline was to run slowly until he was able to drink adequately. Post-operative medication prescribed was: i.m. pethidine 75 mg 4 hourly as required; i.m. metoclopramide (Maxolon) 10 mg as required.

Multiple choice questions *(Answers to Q. 45–53 appear on pp. 72–74)*
The following questions (45–53) are multiple choice questions

45. Mr Williams was to be nursed in the recumbent position for the first four hours after his operation to:
    A. Combat post-operative shock
    B. Reduce haematoma formation
    C. Facilitate nursing observations
    D. Allow easy access for maintaining a clear airway.

46. Which one of following nursing observations are *not* essential during the first 12 post-operative hours?
    A. Recording hourly temperature
    B. Recording the blood pressure and pulse rate frequently and regularly
    C. Checking the movement and sensation of the feet and legs
    D. Observing the volume of drainage and any wound leakage.

47. When turning Mr Williams from side to side immediately after his operation the nurses should instruct him to:
    A. Keep his back straight and roll from side to side with some assistance from them
    B. Do nothing and allow them to lift him onto his side
    C. Lift the upper part of his body by holding his pulley (monkey pole) while they move his legs
    D. Roll around the bed as he wants to.

48. The drug metoclopramide (Maxolon) is prescribed post-operatively to:
    A. Induce sleep
    B. Reduce pain
    C. Increase the blood pressure
    D. Relieve nausea.

During the first night after his operation Mr Williams complained that he was unable to pass urine. He had not passed urine since before his operation and was feeling very uncomfortable. The night nurse tried running the taps to see if this would help him, but with no result, so the surgeon was informed. He told the nurse that she could stand Mr Williams at the bedside and, although this was very painful, he finally managed to pass urine. After this he had no further difficulty micturating.

Five days after his operation Mr Williams commenced mobilization with the aid of a physiotherapist, and he slowly increased the distance which he walked daily. His wound healed well and the sutures were removed on the tenth day after the operation. He then began hydrotherapy and back-strengthening exercises.

---

49. Which of the following are likely reasons for Mr Williams' inability to pass urine?
    A. Acute enlargement of the prostate gland or damage to the sacral nerve roots during the operation
    B. Anaesthetic drugs affecting the parasympathetic nervous system or damage to the genitofemoral nerve during the operation.
    C. Damage to the sacral nerve roots during the operation or the anaesthetic drugs affecting the parasympathetic nervous system
    D. Acute enlargement of the prostate gland or embarrassment at having to use a urinal.

50. When getting Mr Williams out of bed to micturate the nurses should:
    A. Sit him up with his spine straight and swing his legs over the side of the bed
    B. Lift him into a chair at the bedside and stand him up from that position
    C. Turn him prone and swing him across the bed until his legs drop over the side
    D. Roll him into the lateral position at the edge of the bed and sit him up with his legs over the side of the bed.

51. When getting Mr Williams up to walk for the first time, which one of the following instructions is the physiotherapist *unlikely* to give.
    A. Walk keeping the spine erect
    B. Walk with the aid of a walking frame
    C. Avoid sitting
    D. Avoid flexion of the spine.

52. Which one of the following instructions would the physiotherapist give Mr Williams when teaching him the correct method of lifting?
    A. Keep the spine straight and flex the knees and hips
    B. Keep the spine and knees straight and flex the hips
    C. Keep the knees straight and flex the hips and spine
    D. Gently flex the spine, hips and knees.

Sixteen days after his operation Mr Williams was discharged from hospital feeling a little shaky but with no pain in his leg and only a little soreness in his back. An appointment was made for him to see the surgeon in four weeks' time and he was told to attend out-patients' physiotherapy three times a week until then.

---

53. Before he left the hospital Mr Williams should be told to:
    A. Avoid all lifting and rest as much as possible
    B. Walk at least one mile a day and lift only light objects using the method taught
    C. Go for short walks each day and avoid all lifting
    D. Lift light objects only, using the method taught, and go for short walks each day.

Prolapsed intervertebral disc answers

---

1. **True** From the second cervical vertebra to the sacrum the vertebrae articulate with one another anteriorly by partly moveable cartilaginous joints between the vertebral bodies, and posteriorly there are gliding synovial joints between the articulating processes on the neural arches (posterior facet joints).

2. **False** The intervertebral discs are pads of fibrocartilage found between the vertebral bodies. They are part of the cartilaginous joints and their function is to act as buffers or shock absorbers within the spine.

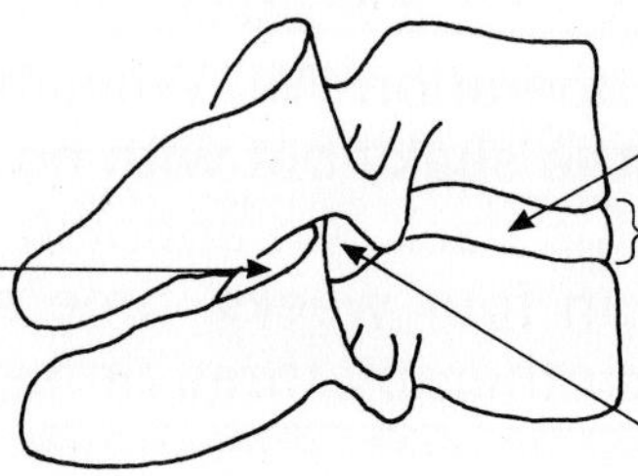

The anterior cartilaginous joint between the vertebral bodies and the posterior synovial joints.

3. **False** The thickness of the discs varies in the different regions of the spine. They are thinnest in the upper thoracic region and thickest in the lumbar region. Overall, they constitute about 1/5th of the length of the spine excluding the first two cervical vertebrae. The proportion of disc to bone is much greater in the cervical and lumbar regions which allows for greater movement in these regions.

4. **True** Each intervertebral disc is not the same thickness throughout. In the cervical and lumbar regions the anterior part of the disc is thicker, which contributes to the anterior convex curves in these regions.

   In the thoracic region the discs are of uniform thickness and it is the shape of the vertebral bodies which makes the curve concave anteriorly.

5. **True** The outer part of the intervertebral disc is the annulus fibrosus, consisting of laminated fibres of collagen and fibrocartilage. Within this lies the nucleus pulposus which at birth is soft and gelatinous but which is gradually replaced by fibrocartilage after about the age of 10 years.

6. **False** Most of the intervertebral disc is avascular except for the most peripheral parts which receive their blood supply from adjacent blood vessels. The avascular parts of the disc get their nutrients by diffusion from the spongy bone of the adjacent vertebrae.

7. **True** In the young adult the intervertebral discs are extremely strong and, providing they are healthy, will only be damaged by a fracture of the vertebral body penetrating the disc. In the cervical region, however, they may be damaged following forced flexion.

8. **False** After about the age of 20 years there is a gradual drying out of the discs and degenerative changes begin to occur resulting in softening and weakening of the annulus fibrosus, and necrosis and sequestration of the nucleus pulposus. The disc may rupture and the nucleus pulposus may herniate through the annulus fibrosus. This usually occurs in the posterior-lateral or the posterior direction, when the posterior ligament may be ruptured; it does *not* protrude anteriorly.

9. **False** In the posterior-lateral type of herniation the protruding nucleus pulposus frequently presses on the adjacent nerve root irritating it and causing referred pain, e.g. sciatica. In a posterior herniation the pressure may be on the dura or, in the lower lumbar region, the cauda equina. Sometimes the disc may be damaged internally by injury without the herniation occurring, and this leads to muscle spasm and pain due to the unequal tension within the joint.

10. **True** Chronic degeneration of the intervertebral discs leads to flattening of the discs, and bony outgrowths (osteophytes) occur along the margins of the vertebral bodies. These changes are referred to as spondylosis.

11. **False** Spondylosis is the result of chronic degeneration of the intervertebral joints (cartilaginous joints). However, this can cause displacement of the posterior facet joints (synovial joints) and lead to osteoarthritis of these posterior joints.

12. **C** In the adult, damage to the intervertebral disc is commonest in the lumbar and cervical regions because there is less bony support for the spine in these areas and most of the movement takes place here. The thoracic spine is supported by the rib cage which reduces the movement, and the vertebrae of the sacrum are fused and with the bony pelvis they form a rigid structure. As most movement takes place in the cervical and lumbar regions they are therefore subject to much greater strain.

13. **D** Prolapse occurs most commonly to the intervertebral disc between the 5th lumbar and the 1st sacral vertebrae. This is because it lies between the mobile lumbar region and the rigid structure of the pelvic girdle and is therefore subject to the greatest strain. When the herniation is posterior-lateral it will frequently cause pressure on the 1st sacral nerve root causing sciatica.

Damage occurs less commonly to the other discs of the lumbar spine and also in the cervical region.

14. **A** When the spine is flexed it is supported by: ligamenta flava, connecting the laminae of adjacent vertebrae; supraspinous ligament, connecting the tips of the spinous processes; interspinous ligaments, connecting the spinous processes; and the posterior longitudinal ligament which lies within the neural canal and is attached to the posterior surface of the bodies of the vertebrae.

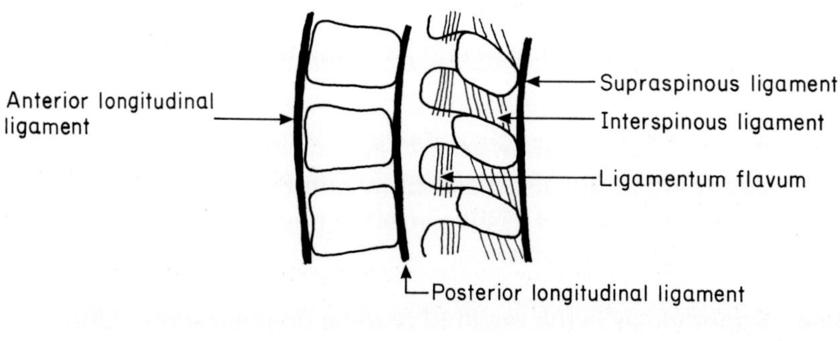

Longitudinal section showing the ligaments supporting the vertebral column.

15. **C** The sciatic nerve is made up of branches of the L4, L5, S1, S2 and S3 nerve roots. It passes through the greater sciatic foramen and through the gluteal region under the gluteus maximus and then down the posterior aspect of the thigh to supply the hamstring muscles (points to be remembered when giving intramuscular injections into the buttocks or the thigh). Finally, it divides just above the popliteal fossa to form the tibial and common peroneal nerves.

16. **False** The intervertebral disc has not slipped out of place but has ruptured. Bed-rest will reduce the movement of the spine and it is hoped that this will relieve the muscle spasm, allowing the inflammation of the ruptured part of the disc and of the nerve root on which it is pressing, to subside. Occasionally, the protruding part of the disc may break off and lie free in the spinal canal.

17. **True** In order to rest the vertebral column in the normal anatomical position Mr Williams should lie on a firm mattress, or if the mattress is soft, a firm board should be placed under it.

18. **False** Sitting on a bedpan for bowel evacuation is likely to aggravate Mr Williams' pain and muscle spasm, and reverse any improvement which he might have had from the bed-rest. If he finds that walking to the bathroom causes a lot of discomfort, a commode should be obtained from the social services department.

19. **True** Providing his pain is not too severe and he avoids bending over the wash-basin, he would probably be allowed to wash and shave while he is in the bathroom. Doing so would cause him less discomfort than attempting to carry out these tasks while he is lying in bed.

20. **True** Indomethacin is an anti-inflammatory drug which will help to reduce the inflammation of the damaged disc and the nerve root where there is pressure.

21. **False** Because indomethacin can cause gastro-intestinal disturbances it should be taken with meals.

22. **True** Indigestion and gastric ulceration are fairly common side-effects of this drug, but sometimes haematemesis may occur without previous gastric symptoms.

23. **True** Headaches, dizziness and lightheadedness occur quite frequently when the drug is first taken but these usually settle if the dose is reduced.

24. **False** Pentazocine is an analgesic drug suitable for moderate to severe pain. For it to be most effective it should be taken when the pain is beginning rather than when it has become severe. It should not be taken more frequently than 4 hourly.

25. **True** Mr Williams should be told not to drink alcohol while taking pentazocine as it may increase the effect of the alcohol.

26. B Limited lumbar movement is most likely caused by muscle spasm around the damaged part of the spine.

27. **C** The common peroneal nerve supplies the tibialis anterior and peroneal muscles which are the muscles that dorsiflex the foot. Damage to the common peroneal nerve causes a drop foot deformity.

28. **D** Straight leg raising is restricted and painful because tension on the nerve is increased as it is stretched over the damaged disc. The pain is increased by dorsiflexing the foot and flexing the neck. Leg raising with the knee flexed is usually unrestricted.

29. **B** Cartilage does not show up on X-ray so the actual disc protrusion would not be seen. If degenerative changes have occurred in the intervertebral disc, narrowing of the disc space may be seen, but this is unlikely as this is the first attack of back pain Mr Williams has had. Associated with narrowing of the disc spaces, osteophytes may be seen, indicating lumbar spondylosis. Of the options given, the only one which could not be excluded from the diagnosis would be a tumour of the nerve root (B).

30. **False** One of the advantages of pelvic traction over simple weight and pulley traction to the legs is that it is not necessary for the patient to lie flat on his back the whole time. Mr Williams could therefore be told that if he finds it more comfortable he can spend periods lying on his side. He should be told that although he is allowed to roll from side to side he should not attempt to sit up. Two pillows only should be placed under his head in order to keep his spine in the normal anatomical position.

31. **True** In order to prevent venous stasis and thrombosis developing Mr Williams should be told to move his legs and feet around as much as possible. Whenever Nurse Little attends to him she should remind him to do this and check that he is doing the exercises properly.

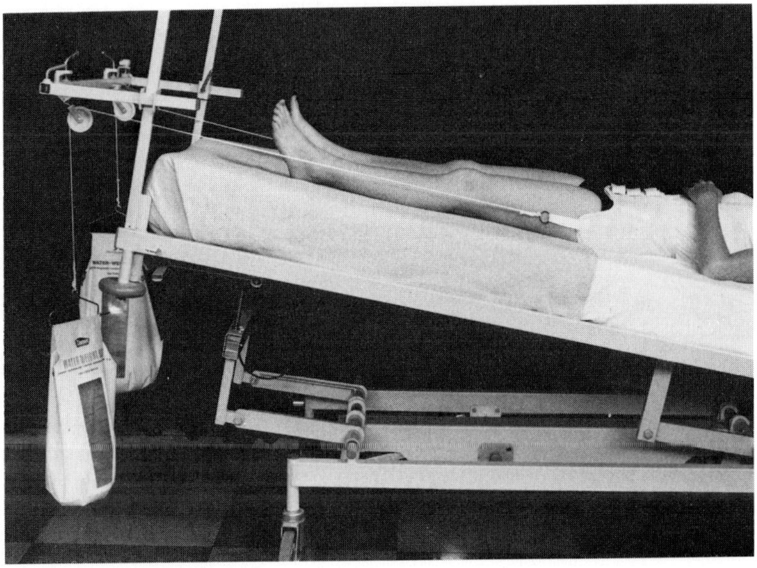

A patient on pelvic traction.

32. **True** The weight of the bedclothes resting on the traction cords would cause friction and thus reduce the efficiency of the traction. A bed-cradle should always be placed in the bed to prevent this friction and also to allow the patient to exercise his legs and feet.

33. **True** If Mr Williams was lying recumbent with the foot of the bed elevated he would not be able to see around the ward. A mirror placed over his bed would enable him to look around and so reduce his feeling of isolation. In addition, he would be able to use it to find things on his locker without attempting to sit up, and with minimal help from the nursing staff he would be able to wash, shave and feed himself.

34. **False** The usual reason for not elevating the foot of the bed at the beginning of the course of traction is to allow the patient a little time to get accustomed to lying in the recumbent position and to wearing a belt around the lower abdomen. Flatulence, indigestion, nausea and constipation frequently occur with this type of traction, but these can be reduced, or even prevented, by allowing the patient a little time to settle before elevating the foot of the bed, even though the traction is not fully efficient during this time. A light diet should be given for the first few days of traction. Bran could be added or a mild aperient given to prevent constipation.

35. **C** A small pillow placed crosswise under Mr Williams' thighs might ease the pain by reducing the strain on his back, particularly during the first few days on traction. It is important that the pillow is placed well up under the thighs so that his hips and knees are slightly flexed, thus reducing the strain on the lumbar spine. The pillow should never be placed under the knees or the calves as this could increase the risk of a deep venous thrombosis developing, and leg movement exercises should still be continued. In addition, analgesia should be given to ease the pain.

36. **D** Mr Williams will need a daily bed bath and, once he is used to the traction, he will be able to do most of this himself with a little help from Nurse Little. In addition, his pelvic belt should be removed, initially three times a day, and the skin under it inspected for soreness. The area should be washed, carefully dried and lightly powdered, and if there is evidence of soreness developing, extra padding could be placed under the belt before it is reapplied.

Accurate recording of fluid intake and output is unnecessary but Nurse Little should give him extra fluids to drink in order to prevent renal stasis, and check that he is passing urine, particularly when he first begins the traction.

Whenever Nurse Little is attending to Mr Williams she should check that the traction is working efficiently. This would include checking that all knots are securely tied and that the cords are running freely over the pulleys and are not fraying. She should make sure that the foot of the bed is elevated and that the weights are correct and are hanging freely.

37. **A** Bran is a natural laxative and should be the one of choice for mild constipation. In addition, Nurse Little should ensure that Mr Williams has a diet which includes plenty of roughage, e.g. wholemeal bread, fresh fruit and vegetables. Sitting out of bed on a commode at the bedside would probably cause Mr Williams less discomfort than sitting on the bedpan but this should only be done with the surgeon's consent.

If a satisfactory bowel action is not achieved by these means then a laxative in oral or suppository form (e.g. bisacodyl) may be prescribed, and the high fibre diet continued.

38. **B** Prior to the radiculography a lumbar puncture is performed. When the examination is to be of the lumbar spine it is usual for the puncture to be made between the second and third vertebrae.

39. **D** A myelogram is the introduction of an oily-based contrast agent (myodil) into the subarachnoid space by means of a lumbar puncture. This is followed by a radiological examination of the spinal canal to diagnose any obstruction of the flow of cerebral spinal fluid by either a tumour or a prolapsed intervertebral disc.

40. **B** A radiculogram is a similar test to a myelogram, using a water-soluble contrast agent, e.g. metrizamide (Amipaque) or iopamidol (Niapam or Omnipaque), and has the advantage of showing the radicles (nerve root sheaths) on the radiographs. It is used to diagnose lesions of the lower lumbar level and demonstrates any compression of the nerve roots.

41. **A** Discography is the injection of a contrast agent (urografin) into the nucleus pulposus of the appropriate intervertebral disc to demonstrate any degeneration or prolapse.

All three examinations could be used to confirm the diagnosis of prolapsed intervertebral disc. Other newer techniques, such as CAT scanning (computerized axial tomography) and lumbar epidural venography, are also available to aid diagnosis in some centres.

42. C Following myelography the patient should rest in his bed for 24 hours with just one pillow under his head. His temperature, pulse and respiration rate and blood pressure should be recorded during this time. The head of the bed should be elevated if the patient complains of a headache or if there are any signs of a reaction to the myodil.

Myodil is not absorbed but remains in the cerebrospinal fluid for many years. Signs of an allergic reaction are nausea, headache, photophobia, pyrexia, general malaise and meningism.

43. E The water-soluble agents used in radiculography have the advantage of being absorbed into the circulation fairly quickly after their introduction. However, some of these substances irritate the spinal cord, so prolonged contact should be avoided.

Following the examination the patient should sit up in a chair for 6 to 8 hours, then lie propped up in bed to 14 to 18 hours. Again, temperature, pulse, respiration rate and blood pressure should be recorded during this time.

After Mr Williams' radiculography, Nurse Little should carry out the above nursing care. In addition, she should tell him not to bend forward to pick things up off the floor, and ensure that he drinks lots of fluid.

Signs of a reaction to the drug are nausea, vomiting and headache.

44. B Except for a mild form of discitis, there are few side-effects following discography. For this reason the patient is encouraged to resume normal activities after the examination.

45. B Mr Williams should be nursed recumbent for the first few hours after his operation so that there is pressure on the wound which will prevent a haematoma forming. His jaw should be held forward while he is unconscious to prevent his tongue falling back and obstructing his airway, and suction apparatus should be at hand to clear his airway if he should vomit.

46. **A** Mr Williams' blood pressure and pulse should be taken and recorded half hourly immediately after the operation; the time can be extended to hourly, then two hourly, as his condition improves (B). Nurse Little should check carefully that the movement and sensation in his feet and legs are normal as the nerve may have been damaged during the operation (C). Any muscle weakness or paraesthesia which was present before the operation will take some time to recover, and it is important that Nurse Little has read Mr Williams' notes and is aware of these symptoms.

Any oozing through the dressing should be noted and a record kept of the drainage in the bottles whenever they are emptied (D). Nurse Little should also note the type of fluid in the drainage bottles, as the presence of clear fluid would probably indicate that there is a leak of cerebrospinal fluid.

It is not necessary to record the temperature hourly unless Mr Williams is shocked or there is a blood transfusion running.

47. **A** Mr Williams should be told to keep his back straight when turning, and with the help of two nurses he should roll gently onto his side. A pillow should be placed behind him to support him in this position and one placed between his knees to prevent pressure. Nurse Little should remove the pillow from between his legs periodically so that he can continue exercising his legs and feet to prevent deep venous thrombosis developing. By about the third day after his operation both this pillow and the one from his back should be removed during the day so that Mr Williams can roll around the bed as he wishes.

The bed should not have a pulley handle on it, as Mr Williams would probably try to use it while turning and in doing so would flex his spine (C). It is not usually necessary for two nurses to lift a patient onto his side following a laminectomy (B), and if it is attempted it is frequently more painful for the patient than if he rolls himself with help.

48. **D** Metoclopramide (Maxalon) is an anti-emetic which could be given if Mr Williams complains of nausea post-operatively.

49. C The action of the anaesthetic drugs on the parasympathetic nervous system may sometimes cause temporary inability to micturate after surgery. In view of the type of operation which Mr Williams has had, irritation of, or damage to, the sacral nerve roots of the pudendal nerve which supplies the external sphincter of the bladder may also cause retention of urine.

50. D When the nurses stand Mr Williams at his bedside it is important that they do this without flexing his spine and without causing him unnecessary pain. This is best achieved by log rolling him to the edge of the bed so that he is lying on his side facing the edge of the bed. His knees and hips are then flexed and his legs gently lowered over the side of the bed. Simultaneously, the nurses assist him into the sitting position while his spine is kept straight and he uses his undermost hand and arm to push up with. He can then be helped into the standing position. He should be supported by two nurses the whole time he is out of bed as pain or the sudden lowering of his blood pressure may cause him to faint. When he is helped back into bed the procedure is reversed.

51. B When Mr Williams starts walking he should be instructed to stand with his back straight (A) and avoid any flexion of his spine (D). He should be told not to sit until after his wound has healed and he should spend his time either walking, standing or lying on his bed. When he is allowed to sit he should sit on a high dining-room type chair with his spine straight and supported; he should avoid so called 'comfortable' sitting-room type chairs which tend to encourage flexion of the spine and bad posture.

52. A In order to prevent further injury to his back when he returns to running his farm it is vital that Mr Williams is taught the correct methods of lifting and how to maintain the correct posture when standing and walking. He should be shown how to keep his back straight when lifting and, by flexing his knees and hips, allow the strain to be taken by the large muscles of the buttocks and thighs.

53. D Mr Williams should be told not to lift heavy objects and if he lifts anything light he should do so using the method taught. He should rest in the recumbent position, either on his bed or on a settee, for periods during the day, and should go for short walks each day making sure he does not go so far that he becomes fatigued. When walking he should strive to maintain a good upright posture and a normal walking gait.

Osteoarthritis of the hip

Miss Ellen Davies is a 64-year-old retired school teacher. She lives alone in a small cottage in the country which she bought several years ago in preparation for her retirement.

When she was working she spent her spare time gardening and walking on the moors with her pet labrador, Ginger, but since her retirement she has found that both these pursuits have become increasingly difficult due to pain and stiffness in her right hip.

She had suffered her pain for some time before she consulted her family practitioner two years ago. He diagnosed osteoarthritis of the right hip and prescribed Distalgesic for the pain and advised her to use a walking stick. An appointment was made for her to see an orthopaedic surgeon.

True/false statements *(Answers to Q. 1–14 appear on pp. 85–87)*
Questions 1–7 are true/false statements relating to the aetiology and pathology of osteoarthritis.

1. The condition only occurs in people over 55 years.
2. Previous injury or disease of the joint may be a predisposing cause.
3. It occurs only in the larger weightbearing joints.
4. Cracking of the subchondral bone which occurs in osteoarthritis is called fibrillation.
5. Eburnation is the term used for the hard shiny appearance of the exposed bony surfaces in advanced osteoarthritis.
6. The bony outgrowths which occur at the edges of the joints are called chondrocytes.
7. Heberden's nodes are bony outgrowths seen on the terminal interphalangeal joints.

Questions 8–14 are true/false statements relating to osteoarthritis of the hip joint.

---

8. Patients with this conditions are often overweight.

9. The pain is aggravated by exercise.

10. The pain does not disturb sleep.

11. The affected leg becomes shorter.

12. The joint becomes flexed, adducted and laterally rotated as the disease progresses.

13. The patient usually walks with an antalgic hip gait.

14. If the right hip is affected the doctor would recommend using a walking stick in the right hand.

When Miss Davies saw the orthopaedic surgeon a month later he confirmed the diagnosis by clinical examination and X-rays. She was found to have 4 cm of shortening of the right leg and she complained to the surgeon that she had difficulty in bending to pick things up off the floor and in putting on her stockings.

The surgeon advised her to continue with her analgesics and prescribed ibuprofen (Brufen) 200 mg to be taken three times a day. He arranged for a raise to be put on to her right shoe and for her to attend a course of out-patient physiotherapy.

Multiple choice questions *(Answers to Q. 15–22 appear on pp. 88–90)*
Questions 15–22 are multiple choice questions.

15. Distalgesic is a compound analgesic preparation containing:
    A. Aspirin, codeine phosphate and caffeine citrate
    B. Dextropropoxyphene hydrochloride and paracetamol
    C. Pentazocine hydrochloride and paracetamol
    D. Dihydrocodeine and paracetamol.

16. The action of ibuprofen (Brufen) is:
    A. Anti-inflammatory and analgesic
    B. Anti-rheumatic and analgesic
    C. Anti-spasmodic and anti-inflammatory
    D. Anti-spasmodic and anti-rheumatic.

17. Which of the following alterations to Miss Davies' shoe would the surgeon most likely order to compensate for the 4 cm of apparent shortening?
    A. 4 cm raise on the heel
    B. 3 cm raise on the heel and 2 cm on the sole
    C. 4 cm raise on the heel and 3 cm on the sole
    D. 3 cm raise on the heel.

18. A heel raise on her shoe would help Miss Davies by:
    A. Making her legs equal in length
    B. Preventing her from limping
    C. Slowing down the progress of the disease
    D. Relieving the strain on her hip.

19. Which one of the following treatments is *unlikely* to be included in the physiotherapy programme?
    A. Straight leg raising exercises
    B. Lying prone with the legs in a neutral position
    C. Short wave diathermy
    D. Hydrotherapy.

20. Regarding Miss Davies' difficulty with bending and dressing, which one of the following actions would be most helpful?
    A. Arrange for a home-help to call daily
    B. Suggest that a neighbour be asked to call in each day
    C. Provide appliances to help her with dressing and other daily tasks
    D. Give her an appointment to attend the occupational therapy department for a full assessment.

Miss Davies' pain improved considerably following her physiotherapy treatment but about a year later she began to notice a gradual deterioration in her hip again. She saw the orthopaedic surgeon who advised her to have a Charnley's total hip replacement, and she was admitted to the orthopaedic ward four months later.

It was arranged that her sister, who lived a few miles away, would look after her dog while she was in hospital, and a neighbour promised to keep an eye on her cottage.

---

21. Before Miss Davies had her operation which one of the following investigations would need to be carried out?
    A. Full blood count, X-rays of chest and pelvis, urine culture, blood grouping and cross-matching.
    B. Urine culture and blood culture, full blood count and X-rays of chest and pelvis
    C. X-rays of chest and pelvis, blood grouping and cross-matching, urine culture and blood culture
    D. Blood grouping and cross-matching, full blood count, blood culture and urine culture.

22. Which one of the following exercises would the physiotherapist teach Miss Davies before her operation?
    A. Breathing exercises, feet exercises and crutch walking
    B. Feet exercises, active exercises of unaffected leg and crutch walking
    C. Active exercises of unaffected leg, feet exercises and breathing exercises
    D. Crutch walking, breathing exercises and active exercises of unaffected leg.

The ward sister allocated Nurse Onions to care for Miss Davies during the period of her operation. In addition to physically preparing Miss Davies for her operation, Nurse Onions carried out a pre-operative assessment specifically to help her plan the post-operative nursing care.

True/false statements *(Answers to Q. 23–31 appear on pp. 90–91)*
Questions 23–31 are true/false statements.

Remembering that the pre-operative assessment is to help Nurse Onions plan the post-operative management, which of the following actions is she likely to carry out? Answer true or false.

23. Weigh Miss Davies and observe her body size.
24. Talk to her to find out if she has any pain or stiffness in any other joints.
25. Test her urine for sugar, acetone, albumen and blood.
26. Ask her about her normal bowel evacuation and whether she takes laxatives.
27. Take and record her blood pressure.

When Nurse Onions prepares Miss Davies for her operation which of the following actions might help to reassure her? Again answer true or false.

28. Attend when the surgeon is explaining the operation to Miss Davies and reinforce what he has said.
29. Tell her that it is not a major operation and that she will soon get over it.
30. Introduce her to another patient who has had the same operation and is recovering well without complications.
31. Show her the X-rays of another patient who has had the same operation.

Early on the morning of the operation Nurse Onions physically prepared Miss Davies for theatre and a premedication of pethidine 50 mg and atropine sulphate 0.6 mg was given at 09.00 hours. At 10.00 hours Nurse Onions accompanied her to the theatre and a right Charnley's total hip replacement was carried out.

Multiple choice questions *(Answers to Q. 32–40 appear on pp. 91–96)*
Questions 32–40 are multiple choice questions.

32. When Nurse Onions prepares Miss Davies for theatre which one of the following lists of tasks is in the most appropriate order?
    A. Assist with a bath and hair wash, cut her toe nails, give an enema or suppository, shave the area of operation
    B. Give an enema or suppository, shave the area of operation, cut her toe nails, assist with a bath and hair wash
    C. Cut her toe nails, give an enema or suppository, shave the area of operation, assist with a bath and hair wash
    D. Shave the area of operation, give an enema or suppository, assist with a bath and hair wash, cut her toe nails.

33. Before giving Miss Davies her premedication Nurse Onions should:
    A. Mark the leg to be operated on and check that the details are correct on the name band
    B. Ensure that Miss Davies has passed urine and ask her to sign the form giving consent for operation
    C. Check that the details are correct on the name band and ensure that Miss Davies has passed urine
    D. Ask Miss Davies to sign the form giving consent for operation and mark the leg to be operated upon.

34. A Charnley hip prosthesis consists of:
    A. A large metal head articulating with a metal acetabular component
    B. A large metal head articulating with a plastic acetabular component
    C. A large metal head articulating with a metal component which screws into the actetabulum
    D. A small metal head articulating with a plastic acetabular component.

After her operation Miss Davies was returned to her bed and was nursed with a triangular pillow between her legs to keep them in abduction. She had a large dressing over her wound and two Redivac continuous drainage tubes draining into bottles attached to the side of the bed.

The ward sister discussed Miss Davies' immediate nursing management with Nurse Onions and stressed the importance of preventing pressure sores developing.

---

35. After this operation it is necessary to nurse the patient with the legs in abduction because:
    A. It relieves the pain by easing the tension on the wound
    B. There is a risk of dislocation when the hip is in adduction
    C. The patient will not be able to move the hip
    D. It keeps the hip in a good functional position for walking.

36. The relief and treatment of the pressure areas of the sacrum and buttocks could best be achieved by:
    A. Removing the abduction pillow and turning Miss Davies onto her left side for pressure area care
    B. Turning her prone for 4 hours a day with the abduction pillow in place
    C. Keeping the abduction pillow in place and easing her on to her left side
    D. Turning Miss Davies from side to side every 4 hours with the abduction pillow in place.

37. When one of the drainage bottles becomes full later in the day Nurse Onions should:
    A. Collect an empty bottle from the sluice area to replace it
    B. Empty the bottle and re-vacuum it before replacing it
    C. Leave it until the other bottle is full, then change them both
    D. Replace it with a sterile bottle which has had the vacuum recharged.

Miss Davies' immediate recovery from her operation was uneventful and on the 4th day after her operation the surgeon said the physiotherapist could stand her out of bed. She could now spend periods during the day with the abduction pillow removed but it must be replaced at night. In addition she should sleep recumbent with just two pillows, and spend and hour each afternoon resting in this position.

Miss Davies complained that she found it very difficult to have a bowel action sitting on a bedpan and the surgeon agreed that she could use a commode at the bedside.

38. When assisting Miss Davies onto the commode Nurse Onions should:
    A. Stay with her all the time she is out of bed
    B. Lift her out of bed with the help of another nurse
    C. Make sure she keeps her legs apart and does not sit upright
    D. Tell her not to put any weight on her right leg.

39. Miss Davies should sleep in the recumbent position with two pillows and spend an hour resting in this position in order to:
    A. Enable her to rest more comfortably
    B. Prevent flexion contracture of the hip
    C. Relieve the pressure on the buttocks
    D. Relieve spasm of her back muscles by constant sitting.

On the 6th day after her operation Miss Davies complained of pain in her right calf muscle. The surgeon diagnosed a deep vein thrombosis and gave her heparin 10 000 iu intravenously, the dose to be repeated every 6 hours for 24 hours. In addition, dicoumarol (warfarin) 50 mg 6 hourly was prescribed.

A prothrombin time estimation was ordered to be carried out daily, and the dose of dicoumarol after the first 24 hours was to be prescribed according to these results.

40. Which one of the following symptoms might Nurse Onions have noticed which might have made her suspect a deep vein thrombosis?
    A. Swelling and blueness of the foot
    B. Pyrexia and whiteness of the foot
    C. Slight pyrexia and swelling of the lower leg
    D. A white foot and no dorsal pedis pulse.

True/false statements *(Answers to Q. 41–52 appear on pp. 96–98)*
Questions 41–52 are true/false statements.

---

41. Prothrombin is a plasma protein.
42. The prothrombin time is shortened when anticoagulant drugs are given.
43. Heparin occurs naturally in the body.
44. Intravenous heparin acts directly on the clotting mechanism.
45. The antidote of heparin is 1% protamine sulphate
46. The action of dicoumarol is to break down the clot.
47. Aspirin should not be given to patients receiving anticoagulants.
48. Patients on anticoagulants should have a full urinalysis daily.

Miss Davies responded well to the anticoagulant therapy and had no complications from her deep vein thrombosis. Two days after its onset she was allowed to continue mobilizing with a supporting stocking on her right lower leg and foot.

By the twelfth post-operative day her wound was healed and the sutures were removed. She was now walking with a pair of elbow crutches and was thrilled by the pain-free movement of her hip and her ability to get about. She spent her days fully dressed, and was able to negotiate stairs and rise from a chair unaided.

Her dicoumarol had been reduced to a maintenance dose of 10 mg twice a day, and on the 16th day after her operation she was discharged from hospital. She went to stay with her sister until she was able to look after herself at home. Out-patient physiotherapy was arranged.

49. Miss Davies should be told to go for a long walks daily to exercise her hip.

50. She should continue resting in the recumbent position for an hour in the afternoon.

51. The physiotherapist should encourage her to progress to taking equal weight on both legs.

52. Once her hip is pain-free she should be told to discard her crutches.

Two weeks later the ward staff had a card from Miss Davies saying that she was continuing to make good progress and had received a wonderful welcome from her dog Ginger. She was looking forward to getting back to her own home shortly and to start looking after her own garden again.

Osteoarthritis of the hip answers

1. **False** Primary osteoarthritis is usually associated with older people but secondary osteoarthritis may occur in younger adults.

2. **True** In secondary osteoarthritis there is a history of previous injury or disease of the joint which has resulted in abnormal mechanical stresses being placed upon it. Such conditions include congenital and growth disorders, such as Perthes' disease, slipped upper femoral epiphysis and congenital dislocation of the hip, which may lead to osteoarthritis of the hip joint. It may also follow such conditions as rickets, Paget's disease, haemophilia, septic arthritis or rheumatoid arthritis.

   In primary osteoarthritis, which is sometimes referred to as ideopathic, there is no such cause, and it is considered to be due to the general degeneration of the joint associated with ageing. There may be contributing factors, such as increased stress on the articulating cartilage, weakness of the cartilage or the poor state of the underlying bone, but the reasons why these should occur are not fully understood.

3. **False** Primary osteoarthritis usually affects one or more of the main weightbearing joints, such as the knees, hips or spine, but it can affect other joints too. There is a generalized type of osteoarthritis which particularly affects women after the menopause, where many joints are affected including the small joints of the hands.

4. **False** 'Fibrillation' is part of the change which occurs in the joint in osteoarthritis. It is the fraying of the articulating cartilage which occurs during the early stages of the disease, not the splitting of the subchondral bone.

   The first visible pathological changes which occur to the structure of the joint are softening and splitting of the articular cartilage. As this progresses the cartilage becomes frayed and ragged — this is termed 'fibrillation' — and the underlying subchondral bone becomes thicker and cracks begin to appear. Cysts then develop in the underlying cancellous bone, due to the increased pressure upon it.

5. **True** When the articular cartilage becomes completely eroded the bony surfaces become exposed in the area of greatest pressure. As the bone degenerates it becomes hardened and appears like polished ivory — hence the expression 'eburnation'.

6. **False** The term used for the bony outgrowths which are seen at the edges of the joints in osteoarthritis is 'osteophytes'. These occur when there is ossification of the unaffected cartilage at the edges of the joints where there is little pressure. These 'osteophytes' can cause restriction of movement of the joints and, when they occur in osteoarthritis of the spine, they may press on a nerve root.

   A 'chondrocyte' is a mature cartilage cell.

7. **True** Heberden's nodes are osseous swellings seen on the dorsal aspect of the terminal phalangeal joints, and are usually part of the more general type of osteoarthritis seen most commonly in women. Bouchard's nodes are similar nodes found over the proximal interphalangeal joints.

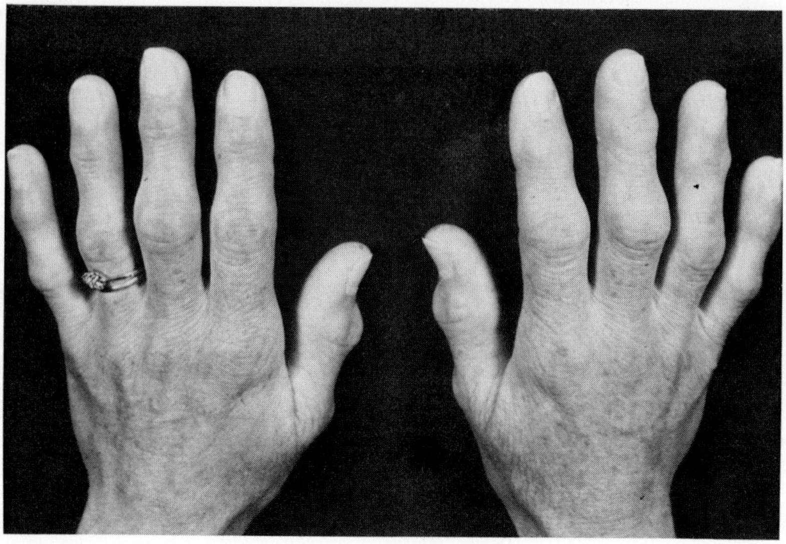

Heberden and Bouchard's nodes.

8. **True** Although many patients with osteoarthritis of the hips and knees are found to be overweight, obesity is not really considered to be an important cause of the condition. However, it does aggravate the condition, and reduction of weight is an important part of the treatment.

9. **True** In the early stages of the disease the pain is worse when movement follows a period of rest. Later, as the disease progresses, the pain becomes more constant.

10. **False** Patients frequently complain that they are woken up by the pain.

11. **False** A patient suffering from osteoarthritis of the hip may think that his leg has become shorter, but this is usually 'apparent shortening' caused by deformity of the hip joint rather than true shortening of the leg.

    To measure the length of the legs the patient should lie in the recumbent position with the anterior superior iliac spines level. 'True shortening' of the leg occurs when there is a difference in length from each anterior superior iliac spine to the tip of each medial malleolus. 'Apparent shortening' is measured from the umbilicus to the tip of each malleolus.

    Congenital abnormalities such as femoral hypoplasia, growth abnormalities such as injury to the epiphyseal cartilage, arthrodesis of the hip or the knee, or a mal-united fracture, may all cause 'true shortening'. 'Apparent shortening' is caused by an adduction deformity of the hip joint.

12. **True** As the disease progresses, stiffness and deformity increase. In the hip joint, flexion and adduction occur with lateral rotation of the leg. It is this deformity which causes the 'apparent shortening'.

13. **True** In order to reduce the stress on the affected joint the patient limps to that side — this is called an antalgic gait. It reduces the pull on the gluteal muscles and thus the force exerted through the hip joint, and so relieves the pain felt on weightbearing on the affected leg.

14. **False** Miss Davies would be told to use the walking stick in the opposite hand to the affected hip, i.e. in the left hand. She should be taught to place the walking stick forward at the same time as she strides forward with her right leg, so taking some of the weight on her stick.

15. B Distalgesic is a compound analgesic of dextropropoxyphene hydrochloride and paracetamol. It is used in the treatment of mild to moderate pain and its potency is similar to codeine but it does not have codeine's constipating effect when used over a long period. Overdosage of Distalgesic, because of the dextropropoxyphene, causes respiratory depression, and liver damage is caused by the paracetemol.

The proprietary names of the other compound drugs mentioned are:

A. Antoin (aspirin, codeine phosphate and caffeine citrate)
C. Fortagesic (pentazocine hydrochloride and paracetamol)
D. Paramol-118 (dihydrocodeine and paracetamol)

16. A The action of ibuprofen is anti-inflammatory and analgesic. Although osteoarthritis is not classed as an inflammatory disease there is often some inflammation present, particularly in the synovial membrane. This is thought to be caused by deposits of bone and cartilage being laid down. Anti-inflammatory drugs do therefore help to relieve some of the painful symptoms.

17. B The usual method of compensating for the 'apparent shortening' is to apply a raise to the heel of the shoe 1 cm less than the measured shortening and a raise to the sole of the shoe 1 cm less than that on the heel. This means that for Miss Davies' 4 cm of 'apparent shortening', a raise of 3 cm would be applied to the heel of her shoe and 2 cm to the sole.

18. D The effect of the alteration to Miss Davies' shoe would be to relieve the strain on her hip. It will not prevent her limping altogether (B), although her limp may not be quite so severe, neither will it have any marked effect on the progress of the disease (C). As her shortening is 'apparent' her legs should theoretically be the same length.

19. A Straight leg raising is an exercise of the quadriceps muscle which is a hip flexor. As there is commonly a flexion contracture of the hip present, it is unlikely to be exercised.

Lying prone (B) would help to correct this deformity, short wave diathermy (C) would help relieve the pain and muscle spasm, and hyprotherapy (D) allows exercises to be performed with much of the body weight eliminated. The warm water would also encourage relaxation and relieve pain.

20. **C** The appliances which Miss Davies would probably find useful would be a 'stocking gutter' and a long shoe horn to help her with dressing. A 'Helping Hand' or similar appliance should be provided to help her pick things off the floor.

Her physiotherapist should be able to organize the purchase of these appliances without the necessity for a full assessment by an occupational therapist (D). Of course, the physiotherapist should teach her how to use them so that she gets full benefit from the appliances when she is at home.

It is unlikely that Miss Davies would need a home help (A), and not really practical for her to ask a neighbour to call in daily (B) to help with such tasks as dressing. It is far better to provide aids so that Miss Davies can be independent at home.

21. **A** Before Miss Davies has her operation her blood should be examined to exclude any disorders, such as anaemia. A full blood count would therefore need to be carried out and her haemoglobin level checked. In addition, her blood group should be identified and her blood cross-matched in preparation for a transfusion during or after the operation.

X-rays of her chest should be taken in order to exclude any disorders or infection of the lower respiratory tract. If there is any evidence of a chest infection this would need to be treated before surgery.

A specimen of urine should be cultured to exclude infection of the urinary tract. Again, if there is any sign of infection this should be treated before the operation takes place.

In view of the fact that a deep-seated wound infection can result in the failure of this operation it is vital that any focus of infection is cleared up before surgery takes place.

22. **C** Teaching Miss Davies to perform particular exercises before her operation would help to prevent post-operative complications occurring.

The following exercises should be included:
- Breathing exercises to prevent post-operative hypostatic pneumonia
- Strong plantar flexion and dorsiflexion of the feet to prevent deep vein thrombosis
- Active exercises of the unaffected leg to prevent stiffness and to strengthen the leg in preparation for mobilization.

Immediately Miss Davies recovers from the anaesthetic she should be encouraged to perform these exercises vigourously.

It is not usual to teach crutch walking before the operation as this is usually easier to learn with the new and more mobile hip in place.

23. **True** By taking note of Miss Davies' weight and body size Nurse Onions will be able to anticipate problems of managing her pressure areas during the post-operative period. There may be particular problems if she is either very thin and bony, or if she is obese.

24. **True** If Miss Davies' other hip or her spine is stiff and painful she may find it difficult to lie in the recumbent position with her legs abducted after her operation. A small pillow placed under her lumbar area might make her more comfortable and possibly a smaller abduction pillow may be needed (see later in the case history). Stiff shoulders may mean that she will not be able to pull herself up with her trapeze to assist with nursing procedures after the operation.

By talking to Miss Davies about her other aches and pains Nurse Onions should be able to predict, and so be prepared for, some of the problems of keeping Miss Davies comfortable after the operation.

25. **False** Her urine should be tested before the operation but this is done to detect any abnormalities present. It would not directly affect Nurse Onions' post-operative management unless such a condition as diabetes mellitus was detected; then regular urinalysis would be required.

26. **True** Prior knowledge of Miss Davies' normal bowel habits will assist Nurse Onions in helping Miss Davies regain a normal bowel action after the operation. It is important to find out whether aperients are normally taken.

27. **False** Although Miss Davies' blood pressure, and also her other vital signs, would be checked before the operation, they would be carried out in order to eliminate abnormalities and would not influence Nurse Onions' post-operative nursing management. However, the results of these tests would be used as a normal baseline when checking the vital signs after the operation.

28. **True** If it is possible, Nurse Onions should attend when the surgeon is explaining the operation to Miss Davies so that she can clarify any queries which may arise later. Any points which the nurse feels she is unable to deal with, or any severe worries which Miss Davies may have, should be referred to the ward sister.

29. **False** A total hip replacement is a major operation and it would be untruthful to tell Miss Davies otherwise. It is the surgeon's responsibility to point out the risks of the operation to her.

30. **True** It would probably help to reassure Miss Davies if she were to talk to another patient who is recovering well from the same operation. However, the patient chosen should be carefully selected as more fear may be created by gory stories.

31. **False** The nurse should not show one patient's X-rays to another patient. In addition, these X-rays are unlikely to be of much help to Miss Davies as she probably would not be able to interpret them.

32. **D** The usual order for the pre-operative preparation is firstly to shave the area of operation and follow this with the bowel preparation. Miss Davies should then be allowed a little time to rest before Nurse Onions assists her with a bath and hair wash and finally cuts her toe nails while they are soft.

N.B. Some surgeons prefer it if their patients are not shaven pre-operatively, and in some centres routine bowel preparation is not carried out. The important point is that, where they are done, both should be carried out before the patient is bathed so that the skin is scrupulously clean before the operation. Skin cleanliness is of paramount importance before this type of operation because of the risk of infection which, should it occur, could lead to removal of the prosthesis and failure of the operation.

33. **C** Before giving her the premedication Nurse Onions should make sure that Miss Davies has passed urine and that all the details are correct on her name band. In addition, she should check that the form giving consent for the operation is signed and that the leg to be operated upon has been marked. It is the surgeon or house officer's responsibility to carry out both of these tasks — never the nurse's.

34. **D** The Charnley's prosthesis has a metal femoral component with a small head which fixes into the intermedullary canal with cement. The acetabular component is made of high density polyethylene and together they form a low friction arthroplasty.

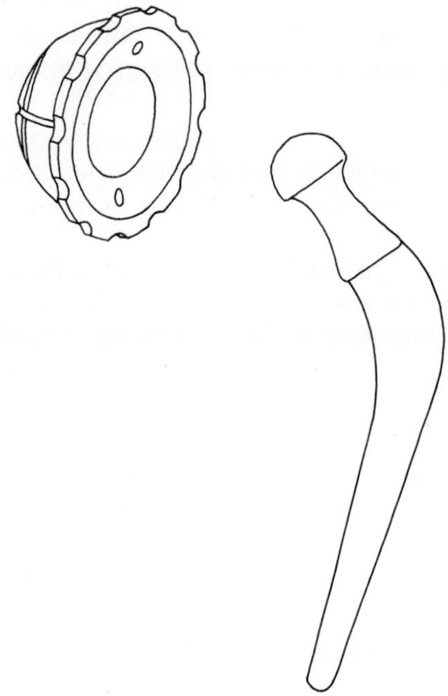

Charnley prosthesis.

Examples of the other prostheses mentioned are:

A. McKee Farrer prosthesis — large metal head articulating with a metal acetabular component.
B. Howse prosthesis — large metal head articulating with a plastic acetabular component.
C. Ring prosthesis — large metal head articulating with a metal component which screws into the acetabulum.

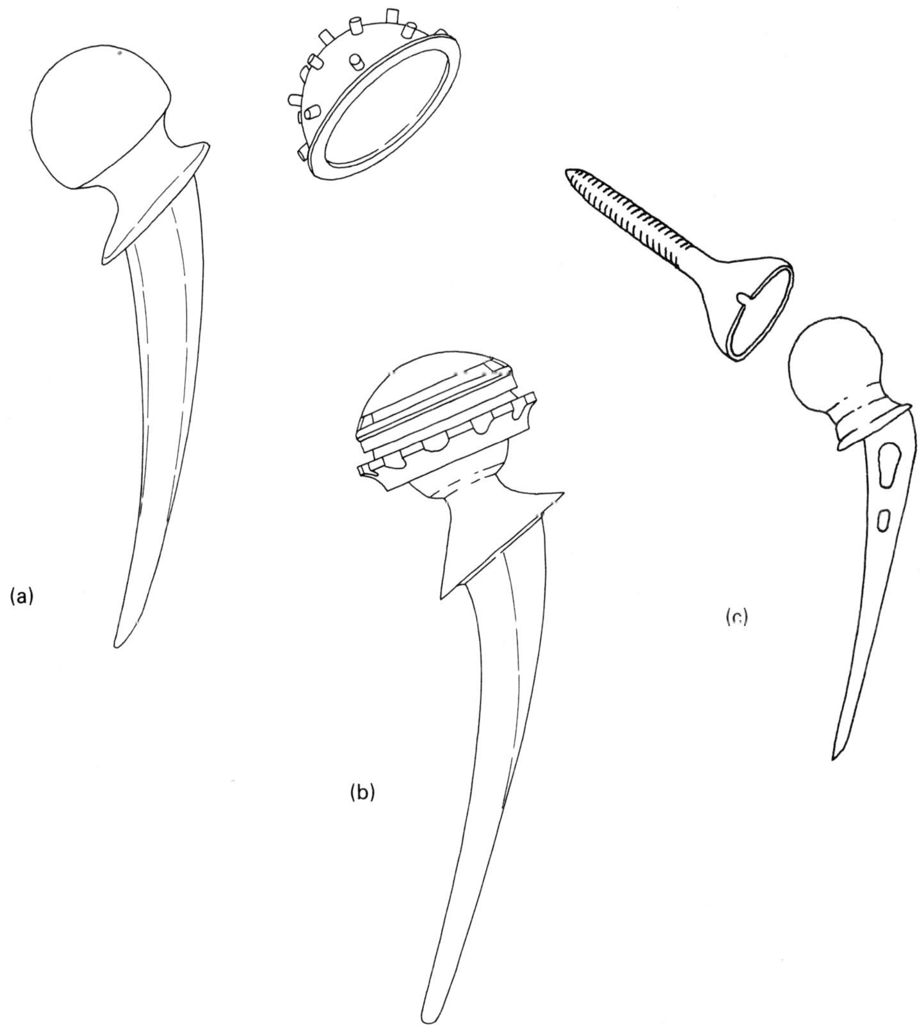

(a) McKee Farrer. (b) Howse. (c) Ring prosthesis.

35. **B** During the operation the greater trochanter is removed with its muscles attached and is wired back into place when the prosthesis has been inserted. In order for this to heal the leg must be kept in abduction for the first one to two weeks. If the leg is allowed to fall into adduction, particularly if the hip is flexed too, there is a considerable risk that the hip will dislocate.

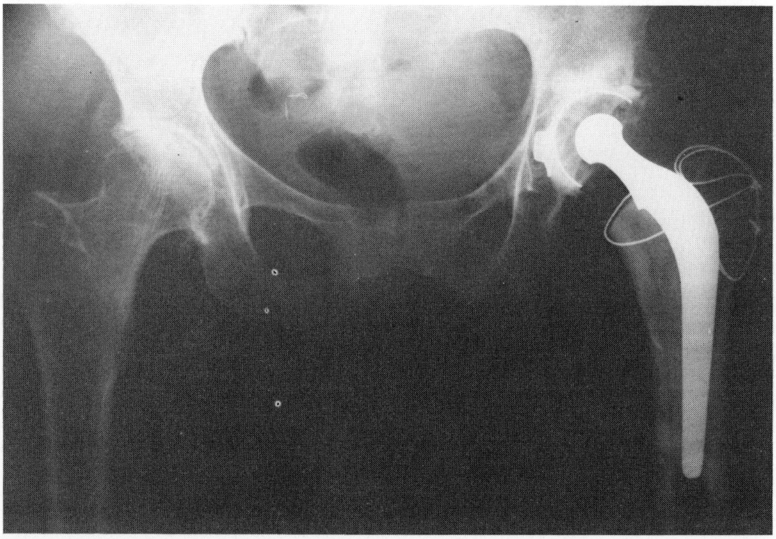

X-ray of Charnley total hip replacement.

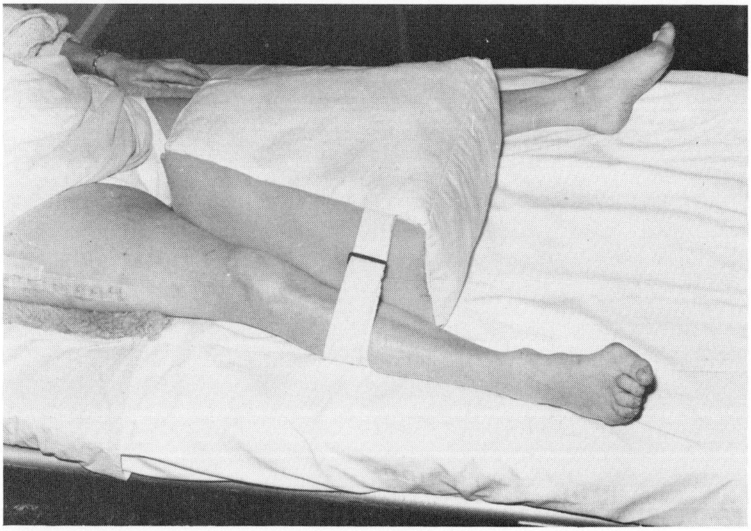

Abduction pillow in position.

36. **C** Miss Davies could either be lifted or rolled onto her left side for treatment of her buttocks and sacral area, but the important point is that the abduction pillow must be kept in place. If soreness begins to develop she could be supported in this position with pillows, or a sheepskin or other appliances may be used to relieve the pressure. Attention should also be given to other areas which are prone to pressure, especially the heels and malleoli.

Because of the risk of dislocating the prosthesis the abduction pillow should not be removed (A), particularly when Miss Davies is turned onto her left side, because her right leg would naturally fall into adduction with the hip in flexion which is the position to be avoided.

It should not be necessary to turn Miss Davies prone (B) unless serious pressure problems develop, necessitating complete relief of pressure for periods of time. The process of turning her into the prone position is likely to cause her considerable pain and distress and, unless very skillfully carried out, could result in dislocation of the prosthesis even with the abduction pillow in place.

Turning Miss Davies from side to side every four hours with the abduction pillow in position (D) would be a reasonable way of relieving the pressure if her buttocks became sore. The main problem with this is that the time she spends lying on her right side is likely to be uncomfortable because of the pain from lying on the operation incision.

37. **D** The bottle must be replaced by a sterile bottle which has had the vacuum created under sterile conditions, preferably in the operating theatre or the sterile supply department. When the bottle is full it must be changed using a sterile procedure, and the tube from the patient should be clamped. A record of the volume of fluid drained should be made.

38. **C** Unless the surgeon orders otherwise, Miss Davies should be able to put a little weight on her right leg and stand at the side of the bed before being lowered onto the commode. However, it is still important that she keeps her legs in abduction when standing and also when sitting on the commode, and that she leans back rather than sits upright. The reason for this is again to prevent the hip dislocating.

39. B If Miss Davies constantly sits upright in bed after the operation flexion contracture of the hip which was present before the operation will tend to increase. In order to correct this, she should spend a period in the afternoon resting on her bed in the recumbent position with just two pillows, and she should sleep in this position at night.

40. C There is usually a slight rise in temperature to about 37.8°C together with some swelling of the ankle when a deep vein thrombosis occurs. The pain in the leg may be quite slight so Nurse Onions should routinely examine Miss Davies' calves and ankles when she is bathing her or making her bed to check for any tenderness or swelling.

Blueness of the foot (A) is not common as the thrombosis only occludes one vein, leaving sufficient vessels patent to carry the volume of blood back to the heart. The presence of a white foot (B and D) and the absence of a pulse (D) indicates an arterial occlusion rather than a venous thrombosis.

41. True Prothrombin is a plasma protein which is produced in the liver and is essential for the clotting of blood. During the clotting process *thromboplastin* (formed when tissues and platelets are damaged), *prothrombin* and *calcium ions* are converted into the enzyme *thrombin*. The *thrombin* changes the plasma protein *fibrinogen* into *fibrin* which forms sticky strands to trap the blood cells and platelets producing the clot.

Damage to tissues and platelets ⟶ thromboplastin

Prothrombin (plasma protein) +
thromboplastin + Ca^{++} ⟶ thrombin

fibrinogen (plasma protein) + thrombin ⟶ fibrin (forms a mesh to trap platelets & blood cells)

The trigger which sets off the whole process is the damage to the tissues and the platelets. In deep vein thrombosis the damage occurs in the vessel walls, caused by degenerative changes and, following surgery or periods of bed rest, compression of the vessels and stagnation of blood.

42. **False** Anticoagulant drugs lengthen the time it takes for the blood to clot. The test usually performed to check the clotting time during anticoagulant therapy is the prothrombin time. This test measures the time it takes for a clot to form when thromboplastin and calcium chloride solution are added to a sample of the patient's plasma. The test is performed on a normal control as well as the blood of the patient receiving anticoagulants.

    Normal prothrombin time is 11–15 seconds.

43. **True** Heparin is a naturally occurring substance which is produced in the liver by the mast cells. It exists in the blood stream side by side with prothrombin but it is not certain that it has any effect on the prevention of blood clotting intravenously. It may play a part in the clearing of fat from the circulation.

44. **True** Heparin injected intravenously acts by directly inhibiting the clotting mechanism by preventing the conversion of fibrinogen to fibrin and also prothrombin to thrombin. Its action is immediate and it prevents the spread of the thrombus, but it does not have any effect in breaking down the clot already formed.

45. **True** The antidote to heparin is 1% protamine sulphate. Because of the risk of bleeding it should be kept readily available when patients are receiving intravenous heparin.

46. **False** Like heparin, dicoumarol does not have any effect on the thrombus already formed, but it acts on the clotting mechanism, thus preventing further clots forming. Its action is to stop the production of prothrombin in the liver and for this reason the effects are not seen for 24–48 hours after oral administration.

47. **True** Aspirin should not be given to patients receiving heparin or dicoumarol because it increases the potency of both these drugs. In addition, there is the risk of gastro-intestinal bleeding in patients on anticoagulant therapy.

48. **False** It is not usually necessary to carry out a full urinalysis daily when anticoagulants are given, but testing the urine daily for blood is a wise precaution in view of the risk of haemorrhage of the urinary tract. Any sign of bleeding from the wound or other source should be reported to the doctor at once so that the appropriate antidote may be given.

49. **False** Only a limited amount of stress should be put on to Miss Davies' artificial hip during the early stages of convalescence; long walks should be avoided. Short walks which do not cause pain or fatigue should be encouraged.

50. **True** By resting on her bed for a period every day, with her hips extended, Miss Davies will aid the healing process and prevent contractures occurring.

51. **True** As Miss Davies' hip becomes stronger she should be taught to take equal weight on both legs while she is still using her crutches.

52. **False** Once she is confident on her crutches and her hip is pain-free she could then progress to two sticks, but only under the supervision of the physiotherapist.

Rheumatoid arthritis

(This case history covers a period of 5 years)

Mary Williamson is 50 years old and lives with her husband Donald and two teenage children in a council house. She had a part-time job as a machinist in a clothing factory and Donald is employed as a bus driver. Her children are 18-year-old Jennifer who is a hairdresser and 16-year-old David who left school six months ago but has not been able to find work.

Five years ago Mary complained of pain and swelling in her joints, especially her wrists and fingers. She later began to have stiffness and pain in her knees, feet and ankles. Her family practitioner diagnosed rheumatoid arthritis and she was sent to the rheumatology clinic at the local hospital.

True/false statements *(Answers to Q. 1–11 appear on pp. 107–108)*
The following questions (1–11) are true/false statements relating to rheumatoid arthritis.

1. Rheumatoid arthritis affects women more frequently than men.
2. It rarely occurs in people under 50 years of age.
3. It is a suppurative type of disease.
4. The disease is thought to be the result of the body producing antibodies which attack the normal cells.
5. In rheumatoid arthritis there is a proliferation of the cells of the synovium.
6. Pannus is the fibrous tissue which replaces the eroded articular cartilage in rheumatoid arthritis.
7. Only joints are affected by the disease.
8. All patients suffering from the disease are found to have the 'rheumatoid factor' present in their blood.

9. Most patients with the disease become severely disabled.

10. Rheumatoid arthritis sometimes begins in women a few weeks after having a baby.

11. The disease tends to run in families.

X-rays and blood tests taken at the rheumatology clinic confirmed the diagnosis. Mary was prescribed a course of ibuprofen (Brufen) and told to rest until the acute pain in her joints had subsided. After a few weeks she was well enough to return to work.

Multiple choice questions *(Answers to Q. 12–24 appear on pp. 108–111)*
The following questions (12–24) are of the multiple choice type.

---

12. The X-rays Mary had taken as an out-patient will:
    A. Confirm the diagnosis beyond doubt
    B. Not show any abnormality at this stage of the disease
    C. Be useful in assessing the progress of the disease
    D. Show severe degeneration of the joint.

13. The test which shows the presence of the 'rheumatoid factor' in the blood is:
    A. Rose Waaler
    B. Kahn
    C. Schick
    D. Coombs'

14. Knowing Mary's diagnosis, which one of the following would most likely be the result of her blood test?
    A. Haemoglobin 12.5 g/100 ml; ESR 12 mm/hour
    B. Haemoglobin 16 g/100 ml; ESR 4 mm/hour
    C. Haemoglobin 20 g/100 ml; ESR 8 mm/hour
    D. Haemoglobin 10.5/100 ml; ESR 20 mm/hour.

15. What type of drug is ibuprofen?
    A. Non-steroidal anti-inflammatory
    B. Corticosteroid
    C. Immunosuppressive
    D. Salicylate.

16. The usual dose of ibuprofen is:
    A. 500 mg daily
    B. 200 mg three times a day
    C. 100 mg twice a day
    D. 50 mg six hourly.

17. In order to reduce the likelihood of side-effects occurring, ibuprofen should be given:
    A. Before food
    B. With food
    C. After food
    D. On an empty stomach.

18. Before prescribing the drug the doctor should check whether Mary suffers from:
    A. Asthma
    B. Heart disease
    C. Diabetes
    D. Hypertension.

19. Which of the following is a side-effect of ibuprofen?
    A. Hypertension
    B. Hepatitis
    C. Agranulocytosis
    D. Indigestion.

20. When telling Mary to rest the doctor would be most likely to tell her to:
    A. Stay in bed all the time
    B. Sit up in a chair during the day
    C. Spend periods of time resting on her bed during the day
    D. Just get up to go to the bathroom.

Over the next four years Mary was seen periodically at the rheumatology clinic. Most of this time she kept fairly well and only had short periods away from work, but six months ago she developed an acute flare-up, with pain especially in her knees, elbows and shoulders.

She now had considerable difficulty walking and, in addition, her hands, wrists and feet were becoming quite deformed. At this stage her problems had become so bad that she gave up her work as a machinist.

She was admitted to the rheumatology ward two months ago for further assessment and treatment. After a full examination plaster resting-splints were made for her hands and legs, and she began a programme of general rest with physiotherapy.

21. When making splints for Mary's hands, her fingers and wrists should be held:
    A. In the position in which they are most comfortable
    B. With any deformities over-corrected
    C. With the deformities corrected within the limits of pain
    D. In the correct anatomical position.

22. The splints should be worn:
    A. At night only
    B. At night and for periods during the day
    C. When Mary's joints are painful
    D. All the time.

23. What action should the nurse take during the night when Mary complained that one of her leg splints was hurting her?
    A. Adjust the splint and reapply it
    B. Remove the splint and place a pillow under her knee
    C. Give her some analgesia
    D. Inform the day staff in the morning.

24. Which of the following points would be most important when applying Mary's splints?
    A. The limbs should be handled with care
    B. The splints must be kept clean
    C. The limbs should be washed, dried and powdered before applying the splints
    D. The circulation of the fingers and toes must be checked.

True/false statements *(Answers to Q. 25–54 appear on pp. 112–119)*
The following questions (25–29) are true/false statements about the deformities and pathological changes seen in rheumatoid arthritis.

---

25. A Baker's cyst is a subcutaneous cyst of the elbow.
26. Ulnar deviation of the fingers causes little dysfunction of the hand.
27. Heberden's nodes are seen on the wrists in rheumatoid arthritis.
28. Dropping of the fingers results from rupture of the extensor tendons.
29. Fixed extension of the knee joints is often the reason for walking difficulty in rheumatoid arthritis.

On admission to hospital the rheumatologist prescribed a course of sodium aurothiomalate (gold salts) for Mary.

The following questions (30–37) are true/false statements about sodium aurothiomalate treatment.

---

30. Sodium aurothiomalate is usually given by intravenous injection.
31. A test dose should be given before starting the course.
32. The usual dose is 50 mg weekly.
33. Most patients show an improvement in their symptoms about a month after starting the treatment.
34. The interval between the injections is usually increased when the symptoms improve.
35. Dermatitis is a rare complication of gold salt therapy.
36. A blood test and urine examination should be carried out at the beginning of the course and after 3 months of treatment.
37. The injection should not be given if the urine protein is 0.3 g/litre.

After two weeks in hospital there was some improvement in Mary's acute pain and she began hydrotherapy and gentle active exercises. She also went to the occupational therapy department for assessment and treatment.

The following questions (38–45) are true/false statements about physiotherapy.

38. Physiotherapy is chiefly concerned with the restoration of function in patients suffering from rheumatoid arthritis.

39. In order to achieve relaxation of the muscles, the water in the hydrotherapy pool is heated to 36°C.

40. Mary should be able to do her own exercises in the hydrotherapy pool.

41. In the hydrotherapy pool, weak muscles can be developed using the resistance of the water.

42. Short-wave diathermy is sometimes used to ease the pain in the active stage of rheumatoid arthritis.

43. Ice packs may be used before the exercises to relieve pain and muscle spasm.

44. Warm paraffin wax is often used before active exercises of the hands or feet.

45. Passive movement exercises should not be performed on patients with rheumatoid arthritis.

The following questions (46–49) are about occupational therapy.

46. One of the occupational therapist's chief aims is to prevent Mary becoming bored while in hospital.

47. The occupational therapist should carry out a functional assessment at the start of Mary's treatment.

48. Any self-help aids which might help Mary perform particular tasks should be provided.

49. An assessment of Mary's personality and mental state would not normally be carried out.

Over the following weeks Mary showed a gradual improvement in her condition. Her joints became less painful and even though she had considerable deformities in her hands and stiffness in her shoulders, elbows and knees, she was now able to get about with the aid of a walking frame. With the aids provided she became much more independent and was able to deal with her own personal hygiene and to dress herself.

During this time the physiotherapist and occupational therapist visited Mary's home and suggestions were made about modifications which they thought would be helpful. A downstairs toilet and shower were built and Donald converted the dining room into a bed-sitting room so that there would be no need for Mary to go upstairs.

Twelve weeks after she was admitted Mary was discharged home. She had an appointment to attend the out-patient clinic in four weeks and transport was arranged for her to attend out-patient physiotherapy three days a week. Arrangements were made for the community nurse to call in to give Mary her injections of sodium aurothiomalate.

The following questions (50–54) are true/false statements.

50. Aids to help Mary dress herself are provided free of charge.

51. Mary's walking aid would be lent to her for the period of time she needed it.

52. Mary would not be eligible for a home help because she lives with her husband and family.

53. Mary's family would have to pay for the alterations to the house themselves.

54. Even though a bedroom and bathroom have been made downstairs for Mary, she should be told to try to walk upstaris periodically so that she does not lose the ability to do so.

Rheumatoid arthritis answers

---

1. **True** In the United Kingdom the incidence of rheumatoid arthritis in women is 6% and 2.5% in men. This increases to 6% in men over 75 years and 16% in women over 65 years.

2. **False** It can start at any age but the onset is commonest between the ages of 35 and 55 years.

3. **False** It is a chronic inflammatory disease which does not produce pus.

4. **True** The cause of rheumatoid arthritis is unknown but it is evident that a person with the disease develops an auto-immune reaction where antibodies are produced which attack the normal cells. Much research is being carried out into why this change occurs in the immunological response. One theory is that an infective agent, such as a virus, may be the cause, but no definite organism has yet been identified.

5. **True** The disease primarily affects the joints, and it begins with inflammatory changes in the synovial membrane. The normal single layer of cells which forms the synovial membrane proliferates and becomes swollen, vascular and several layers thick. It spreads over the articular cartilage by forming tongue-like projections or villi, which adhere to the margins of the cartilage. The cartilage is replaced by fibrous tissue infiltrated with chronic inflammatory cells.

6. **True** The tissue which is produced by the erosion of the articular cartilage is called pannus. As the disease progresses the underlying bone also becomes eroded and replaced by pannus, and it may even extend to the subchondral bone to form cysts.

7. **False** Although the disease chiefly affects the joints, other tissues and organs may be involved, possibly due to the spilling over of the immune complexes into the circulation. There is often inflammation of the tendon sheaths which may lead to tendons rupturing. Muscles become wasted and osteoporosis is common. Subcutaneous nodules may develop and rheumatoid nodules may be found in the heart, lungs and eyes. Arteritis may occur and the peripheral nerves may be affected by vasculitis. This widespread systemic disease is sometimes referred to as 'rheumatoid disease'.

8. **False** About 70% of patients suffering from the disease are found to have the antibody known as the 'rheumatoid factor' present in their blood. It is also present in about 5% of unaffected people and can appear during other chronic diseases such as tuberculosis, hepatitis or bacterial endocarditis. For this reason it cannot be used to confirm the diagnosis.

9. **False** Although the course of the disease varies considerably in individuals, the general picture is one of periods of exacerbation, where the patient is generally unwell, followed by periods of remission. Only a small percentage (about 10% of those diagnosed) progress to complete disability; about 20% have no further problem after a short episode of arthritis; and the remainder continue with the disease for many years with variable amounts of disability.

10. **True** The onset of rheumatoid arthritis is sometimes precipitated by stress and it may begin shortly after a woman has a baby. In established rheumatoid arthritis it is usual for a remission to occur during the pregnancy but this is often followed by a period of exacerbation after the birth of the baby.

11. **True** There is a higher incidence of confirmed rheumatoid arthritis in families than in controls but heredity is not generally considered to be an important factor in the cause of the disease.

12. **C** During the early stages of the disease the X-rays are only likely to show soft tissue swelling. Later, as the disease progresses, they will show any erosion of bone and deformity. Their value will therefore be in assessing the progress of the disease.

13. **A** The Rose Waaler or sheep cell agglutination test (SCAT) is one of the tests which demonstrates the presence of the 'rheumatoid factor' in the blood. Other tests are the latex factor and the rheumaton test, but, as previously stated, not all patients with rheumatoid arthritis have the rheumatoid factor present in the blood.

Kahn reaction (B) is a blood test used in the diagnosis of syphilis, Schick test (C) is a skin test used to ascertain whether a person is susceptible to diphtheria, and Coombs' test (D) is a blood test which tests for the presence of antibodies coating the red cells and is positive in haemolitic disease of the newborn and in acquired haemolitic anaemia

14. **D** Patients suffering from rheumatoid arthritis are usually anaemic and have a raised ESR. Of the options given (D) has a low haemoglobin (normal 12–18 g/100 ml) and a raised ESR (normal 1–13 mm/hour.)

The type of anaemia which is seen in rheumatoid arthritis is that of a chronic infection, i.e. there is a slightly reduced haemoglobin (Hb) and mean corpuscular haemoglobin concentration (MCHC), a low serum iron and a low iron-binding capacity.

The erythrocyte sedimentation rate is an indicator of the amount of inflammatory activity taking place, and this is usually raised during the active stages of the disease. The level may be normal during the early or inactive stages and also during treatment with systemic corticosteroids, gold or penicillamine. It is therefore not a diagnostic test but is used to monitor the amount of inflammatory activity taking place.

15. **A** Ibuprofen is a non-steroidal anti-inflammatory drug which has analgesic properties. It is one of the drugs which may be used to relieve pain and reduce inflammation in rheumatoid arthritis and can be used as an alternative to salicylates (aspirin) (D) which have more gastric side-effects.

Because of the very serious side-effects of corticosteroids (cortisone, prednisone, prednisolone) (B), they are only used in very severe cases of rheumatoid arthritis where non-steroidal anti-inflammatory drugs have failed to control the progress of the disease. Frequently, the patient develops a tolerance to these drugs and it becomes necessary to increase the dose which often leads to the development of the features of Cushing's syndrome.

Immunosuppressive drugs (cyclophosphamide, chlorambucil) (C) may very occasionally be prescribed in very severe rheumatoid disease where non-steroidal or steroidal anti-inflammatory drugs have failed. Because of the very serious side-effects (i.e. bone marrow suppression) they are used with extreme caution.

16. **B** The usual dose of ibuprofen is 200–400 mg three times a day.

17. **C** Whenever possible it should be given after meals as this reduces the likelihood of gastric irritation.

18. **A** Non-steroidal anti-inflammatory drugs should be used with caution in patients suffering from gastro-intestinal conditions, allergic conditions such as asthma, and disorders of the kidneys or liver. It is therefore important to obtain a detailed history from the patient before prescribing the drug.

19. **D** Generally speaking, the side-effects of this drug are fairly mild, but they do include gastric irritation, nausea, rashes, vertigo and hearing disturbances. It is important that the nurse observes a patient who is receiving this drug for any of these symptoms.

20. **C** Mary would most likely be told to get up and move about during the day in order to prevent stiffness occurring. She should spend periods of the day resting on her bed and she should be told about the importance of resting with her joints in a good functional position in order to prevent deformities developing. For example, she should be told not to curl up on her bed or to lie on her back with a pillow under her knees as both these positions can lead to the development of flexion contractures of her hips and knees.

21. **C** The function of the splints is to allow the hands and wrists to rest in a comfortable position which also prevents further deformity developing. This usually means that some of the deformity is corrected when the splint is made but painful over-correction should be avoided.

22. **B** The times when the splints are to be worn should be decided by the doctor. The usual practice during the sub-acute stage of the disease is for the splints to be worn at night and during rest periods during the day. When the splints are not being worn, gentle exercises are usually done to prevent stiffness occurring.

During an early acute phase of the disease or a period of acute exacerbation, a period of complete bed-rest may be ordered. The splints would probably then be worn all the time and just removed for washing the skin and perhaps wax baths for the hands. Nursing and physiotherapy staff should ensure that the correct position is maintained in bed, and the physiotherapist should give breathing exercises and static quadriceps exercises with the leg splints on.

23. **A** If the splint is uncomfortable it should be removed and adjusted before it is re-applied, in an effort to make it more comfortable. If the discomfort persists, the splint should be removed and the leg supported in a comfortable position. A pillow must not be placed under the knee (B) as this will lead to an increase in the flexion contracture deformity commonly seen in rheumatoid arthritis. If the cause of Mary's pain is joint pain then analgesia should be given as prescribed (C) once the splint has been made comfortable. The day staff should be told about the problems with the splint the next morning (D) so that adjustments can be made to the splint or possibly a new splint provided if the problem arises again.

It must be stressed that all resting splints must be comfortable and any discomfort from the splint must be dealt with promptly and effectively. A person with rheumatoid arthritis has enough pain from her arthritis without the added discomfort of a badly fitted or applied splint.

24. **A** Of the options given, careful handling of the limbs is the most important. As well as being painful when handled, the joints are liable to subluxation or dislocation, and if the bones are osteoporotic they may fracture. In addition, the skin becomes friable and bruises easily in advanced rheumatoid arthritis.

The splints should be kept clean (B) and should never be applied so tightly that the circulation to the fingers or toes is impaired (D). It is not necessary to wash the limbs each time the splints are removed (C). It should be sufficient to wash the limbs daily when Mary has her bath. At this time the skin should be examined for any signs of soreness, and carefully dried before the splints are reapplied.

25. **False** A Baker's cyst is a fluid-filled bursa which occurs in the popliteal space behind the knee, and is usually associated with rheumatoid arthritis or osteoarthritis. It is comprised of a herniation of synovial membrane which is usually connected with the knee joint. Occasionally it may extend down between the calf muscles causing acute pain which resembles thrombophlebitis.

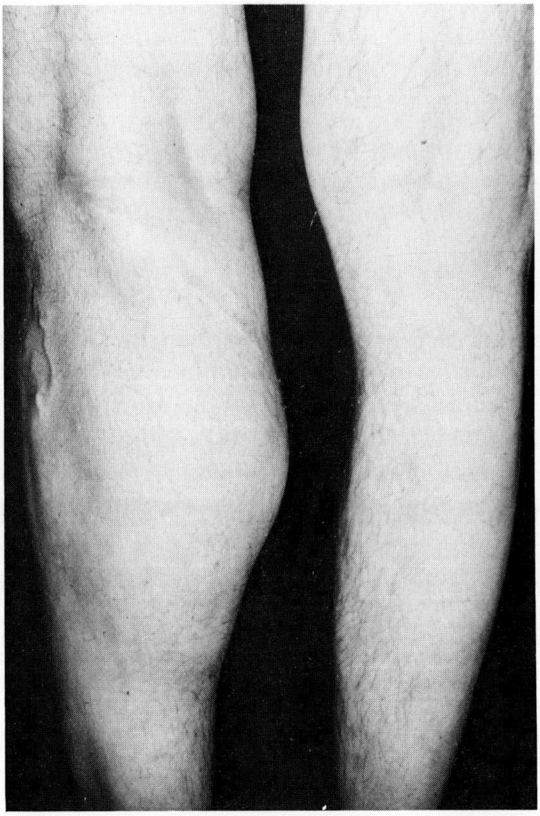

Baker's cyst.

26. **True** In advanced rheumatoid arthritis ulnar deviation of the metacarpophalangeal joints is fairly common, but, although the deformity may be severe, the effect on the function of the hand is often only slight.

The ulnar deviation is usually associated with anterior subluxation of the metacarpals on the phalanges and medial dislocation of the extensor tendons.

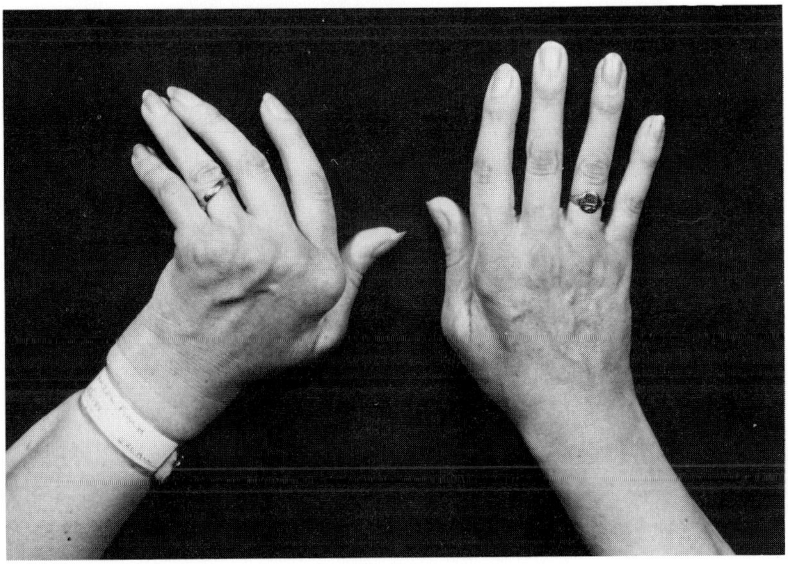

Ulnar deviation of the fingers.

27. **False** Heberden's nodes are osseous swellings which are sometimes found on the dorsal aspect of the terminal phalangeal joints of patients with osteoarthritis, not rheumatoid arthritis. Bouchard's nodes are found over the proximal interphalangeal joints.

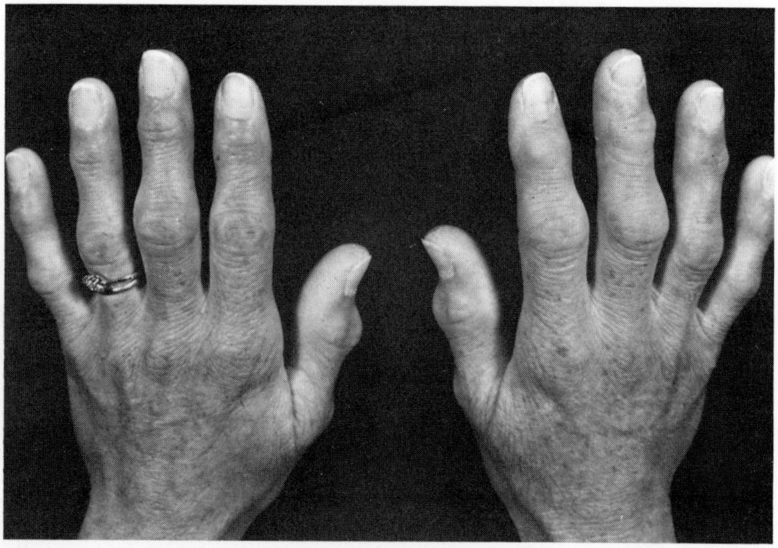

Heberden's and Bouchard's nodes seen in osteoarthritis.

28. **True** In advanced rheumatoid arthritis the extensor tendons may rupture. This results in dropping of the affected fingers. Other finger deformities such as 'swan neck' deformity (hyperextension of the proximal interphalangeal joint and flexion of the terminal interphalangeal joint), 'trigger fingers' (caused by nodules in the flexor tendons) and overriding of the fingers, lead to considerable loss of function and power in the hands.

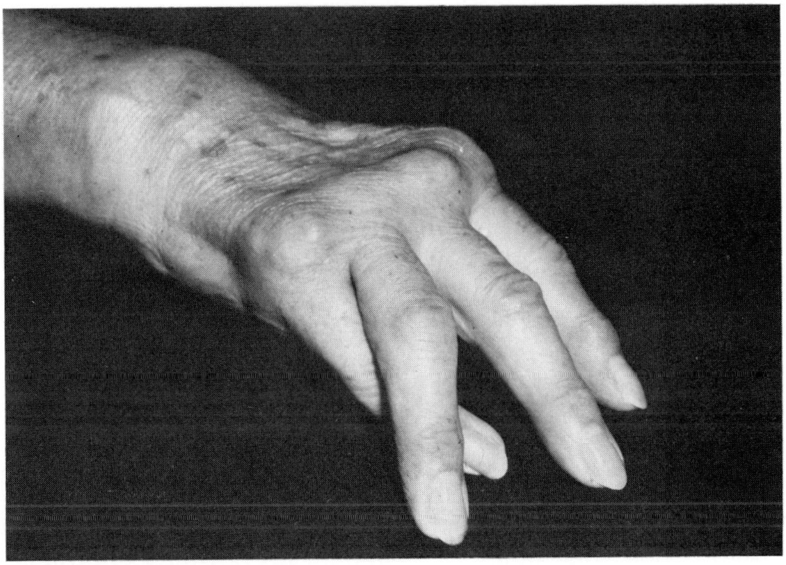

Overriding of the fingers.

29. **False** In rheumatoid arthritis the common deformity of the knees is flexion contracture with a valgus, or less commonly a varus, deformity too.

30. **False** Sodium aurothiomalate (gold salts) is given by intramuscular injection, and the injection should be given at a different site each time so that the danger of local irritation is reduced.

31. **True** A test dose (usually of 10 mg) is given at the beginning of the treatment to test for any reaction to the drug.

32. **True** Some doctors gradually increase the dose until the patient is receiving 50 mg weekly, while others immediately begin á course of 50 mg weekly after a test dose. The course usually lasts 20 weeks (1 g total).

33. **False** The effect of the treatment usually takes several weeks and it is not until the patient has received about eight 50 mg doses that there is any improvement in the symptoms.

34. **True** When there is an improvement in the symptoms the interval between the injections is usually then gradually increased to two weekly, then four weekly or even six weekly. If a relapse occurs the dose can be increased to 50 mg weekly again.

35. **False** The principal side-effect of gold salt treatment is dermatitis. This can be severe and exfoliative, so nurses should be particularly vigilant when caring for a patient who is receiving this type of treatment.

Other side-effects include blood disorders such as thrombocytopenia, agranulocytosis and leucopenia, and damage to the kidneys and the liver.

36. **False** In order to recognise early bone marrow damage causing blood disorders, a full blood count should be carried out either before each injection or at regular intervals during the course. Similarly, the urine should be tested for the presence of protein which would indicate renal damage.

The gold binds to the plasma protein in the blood and concentrates in the kidneys where severe damage can occur because the excretion is slow. At the end of the course of injections there is a high reserve in the system which may take as long as a year to eliminate.

37. **True** Usually, the level of proteinurea at which the drug is omitted is 0.3 g/litre. When an abnormality is found in the blood or the urine test, the doctor must be informed and he will decide whether the treatment should be discontinued.

38. **True** Physiotherapy in rheumatoid arthritis is concerned with assessing the patient's physical ability and in improving the function and mobility of the affected joints. In order to accomplish this, pain and stiffness must be relieved and weak muscles strengthened. This is achieved by exercises which are frequently preceded by the application of heat and/or cold and sometimes by the use of hydrotherapy.

39. **True** The water is heated to body temperature which gives the patient a general feeling of well-being and relaxes the muscles.

40. **False** Mary should be closely supervised all the time she is in the pool. The warm water will support the limbs, enabling exercises to be carried out with greater ease and less pain, but the physiotherapist should be there to instruct and supervise.

Many handicapped people feel very anxious about going into the water so it is important to gain their confidence before starting the treatment, as a person with a real fear of the water will not benefit from the treatment.

41. **True** The water in the hydrotherapy pool supports the body and the limbs, giving the person a feeling of weightlessness which helps movement. In addition, the limbs can be exercised against the resistance of the water thus strengthening weak muscles.

42. **False** In short-wave diathermy high frequency electrical currents are passed through the tissues and converted into heat. This causes vasodilation, and, because rheumatoid arthritis is an inflammatory condition, short-wave diathermy is not suitable for use during the active stages of the disease when the tissues are inflamed.

43. **True** The application of cold by means of an ice pack before exercises are carried out is often effective in reducing muscle spasm and relieving pain. The effect of the cold pack is to cause superficial vasoconstriction which is followed by vasodilation. It is particularly successful for a joint which is inflamed.

Likewise, warm packs may be applied over a painful joint before it is exercised, for example the shoulder joint. Warmpacks are popular with many patients because they seem to give great relief from pain.

Whether ice packs or moist warm packs are applied, it is important to avoid burning the skin. Skin sensation should be tested before the pack is applied and the patient told to inform the nurse or physiotherapist immediately if discomfort is felt.

44. **True** Paraffin wax at body temperature may be applied to stiff or painful hands or feet and then they are wrapped in a towel or polythene bag. When the wax is cool it is removed and the patient can mould it into shapes and thus exercise the hands.

45. **False** Rheumatoid joints which do not function may be gently put through a range of passive movements in order to maintain movement and to prevent contractures developing.

46. **False** Like the physiotherapist the occupational therapist's aim is to improve the patient's joint function and general mobility, but unlike the physiotherapist she is chiefly concerned with the function of the whole limb or whole body rather than individual muscles or joints. The occupational therapy is geared towards retaining or regaining as much personal independence for the patient as possible.

While Mary is spending long periods resting in bed she may need extra facilities to help her pass the time, e.g. a book stand to support her book, but providing diversions for her is only a very small part of the occupational therapist's role. Once Mary begins her programme of occupational therapy and physiotherapy she will have little time to become bored.

47. **True** An assessment of Mary's ability to carry out activities of daily living is undertaken at the beginning of the course of occupational therapy. This should include an assessment of how well she is able to look after herself (i.e. dressing, bathing, using the toilet and feeding herself). In addition, she should be assessed in the occupational therapy kitchen to see how well she can prepare and cook food herself.

48. **False** Self-help aids such as long-handled eating utensils, a raised toilet seat or special kitchen gadgets can certainly be provided but not just because they might be helpful. Before any aids are supplied it is important that the occupational therapist and Mary feel that each aid enables her to perform a particular task with greater ease. Any aid supplied which is not of benefit to the patient, or whose application is unclear, is likely to be discarded.

49. **False** It is important to assess the patient's psychological state and the degree of motivation which she possesses for the treatment to be successful. Unless this is done, a patient who responds well while in hospital may return home and become completely dependent on her family and lose the independence which she had achieved in hospital.

It must be stressed that Mary's successful rehabilitation will depend upon the joint efforts of all who are involved with her care: these include the rheumatologist, the nurses, the physiotherapist, the occupational therapist, the medical social worker and her family. It is important that there is communication between members of the team so that each can help the work of the other to Mary's benefit, e.g. the nurses can help and encourage Mary to use any appliances which have been provided by the occupational therapist.

50. **False** Simple aids such as those used for dressing are usually bought by the patient.

51. **True** Walking aids and crutches are usually provided free by the hospital authorities, and the patient is usually asked to sign a form undertaking to return them when they are no longer needed.

52. **False** Any patient who is chronically sick or handicapped is eligible for a home help if it is considered that she needs one. The home help would be organized through the social services department before Mary leaves hospital and it is usual for the patient to be charged for the service.

53. **False** Provided permission to carry out the alterations to the house has been obtained from the social services department, the local authority would then pay a part or all of the cost.

54. **False** If Mary finds going up and down the stairs difficult, forcing herself to do so would be of little value and, indeed, may cause further damage to her diseased joints.

Fractured neck of femur

Mrs Betty Dyke is 82 years old and lives with her 90-year-old husband, Don, in a terraced house. Mr Dyke suffers from arthritis and for the past year he has been a little confused and unsteady on his feet. Mrs Dyke is rather deaf and, although she is small and looks frail, she keeps fairly fit for her age.

Mr and Mrs Dyke are both very independent. Mrs Dyke has managed to look after her husband at home with the help of the community nurses who come in twice a week. They both go to the local day hospital on Mondays and Fridays and on the other days they receive 'meals on wheels'. They have a home help three days a week and their son and daughter-in-law, who live in a small flat a few streets away, call in most days to see them.

During the past winter the health visitor and the community nurses have been concerned about the welfare of the elderly couple. The only form of heating in the house is a coal fire and this is always small as Mrs Dyke is reluctant to make a bigger fire because of the cost of fuel. The health visitor has been trying to persuade them to give up their home and move to 'sheltered accommodation' but they have both resisted this vigorously. They cannot live with their son because the flat is too small.

Matters came to a head one day in April when Mrs Dyke was putting out the milk bottles. She tripped on the doormat and fell heavily onto her right side. She tried to get up but could not because of the severe pain in her right hip. Fortunately, the community nurse called a few minutes later to bath Mr Dyke and found Mrs Dyke lying by the front door in a state of shock and with her right leg twisted under her. The nurse thought she had fractured her hip.

Multiple choice questions *(Answers to Q. 1–4 appear on pp. 130–131)*
The following questions (1–4) are multiple choice questions.

---

1. Which one of the following actions should the nurse take first?
   A. Phone for an ambulance
   B. Cover Mrs Dyke with a blanket
   C. Move Mrs Dyke on to her bed
   D. Apply a splint to Mrs Dyke's leg.

2. Which of the following signs would indicate to the nurse that Mrs Dyke was suffering from shock?
   A. Slow pounding pulse, flushed face and extremities, and low blood pressure
   B. Rapid feeble pulse, cold pale face and extremities, and raised blood pressure
   C. Rapid feeble pulse, flushed face and extremities, and raised blood pressure
   D. Rapid feeble pulse, cold pale face and extremities, and low blood pressure.

3. The kind of shock which Mrs Dyke was suffering from would be described as:
   A. Oligaemic
   B. Toxigenic
   C. Neurogenic
   D. Anaphylactic.

4. How should the nurse treat Mrs Dyke's shock while she is waiting for the ambulance to arrive?
   A. Hold her hand and reassure her by chatting to her
   B. Give her and Mr Dyke a cup of tea
   C. Raise her feet onto pillows to allow the blood to circulate to the vital organs
   D. Cover her with blankets and give her a drop of whisky to warm her.

Mrs Dyke was very worried about having to leave her husband. The nurse telephoned her daughter-in-law, Mary and also the family doctor, to see what arrangements could be made for Mr Dyke. Mary, arrived just before the ambulance and promised to stay with Mr Dyke until the doctor arrived. She tried to console her mother-in-law and told her that as soon as she had any news she would come around to the hospital to tell her.

When Mrs Dyke arrived at the accident and emergency department she was examined fully and X-rays were taken. These showed that she had a right sub-capital fracture of the femoral neck.

True/false statements *(Answers to Q. 5–11 appear on pp. 131–132)*
The following questions (5–11) are true/false statements.

5. Fractures of the neck of the femur are commoner in women than in men.
6. It is probable that Mrs Dyke has osteoporosis which would cause the neck of the femur to fracture with minimal force.
7. A sub-capital fracture is extracapsular.
8. Avascular necrosis of the head of the femur is a complication of an intertrochanteric fracture.
9. Sub-capital fractures of the femur do not have a good capacity for healing.
10. The rate of healing of a sub-capital fracture may be delayed by the synovial fluid in the joint.
11. Following a fracture of the neck of the femur the leg lies in medial rotation.

The surgeon explained to Mrs Dyke that she would need an operation on her hip in a few days time, and that in the meantime traction would be applied to her leg to make it more comfortable.

Nurse Davies had been assigned by the ward sister to care for Mrs Dyke when she came to the ward, and the nurse prepared a bed to be taken to the accident and emergency department. The surgeon instructed Nurse Davies to apply Hamilton Russell traction to Mrs Dyke's right leg.

Multiple choice questions *(Answers to Q. 12–26 appear on pp. 133–138)*
The following questions (12–26) are multiple choice questions.

12. When preparing the bed for Mrs Dyke, Nurse Davies should ensure that it has a:
    A. Variable height adjustment, Balkan beam attachment and trapeze or 'monkey pole'
    B. Balkan beam attachmant, trapeze or 'monkey pole' and back-rest
    C. Trapeze or 'monkey pole', firm mattress and back-rest
    D. Firm mattress, variable height adjustment and back-rest.

13. When applying Mrs Dyke's Hamilton Russell traction Nurse Davies should:
    A. Apply above-knee extensions, place a sling under her knee and elevate the foot of the bed
    B. Apply below-knee extensions, place a sling under her knee and nurse her with two pillows under her head
    C. Apply below-knee extensions, place a sling under her knee and elevate the foot of the bed
    D. Apply above-knee extensions, elevate the foot of the bed and nurse her with two pillows under her head.

14. The most suitable method of applying the Hamilton Russell traction to Mrs Dyke's leg would be:
    A. Ready-made sideways-stretch strapping extensions
    B. Foam-backed non-adhesive extensions
    C. Steinmann's pin
    D. Denham pin.

15. Hamilton Russell traction is a type of:
    A. Fixed traction
    B. Balanced traction
    C. Manual traction
    D. Intermittent traction.

16. Remembering that Mrs Dyke is rather small and frail which one of the following weights should Nurse Davies apply to her traction?
    A. 2 kg
    B. 2.5 kg
    C. 3.5 kg
    D. 4 kg.

17. Mrs Dyke should have an operation on her hip because:
    A. The fracture will not heal without internal fixation, and complications may arise if she spends a long period in bed
    B. A long stay in hospital would result in her becoming dependent on others, and she was anxious to get home quickly to look after her husband
    C. The fracture will not heal without internal fixation, and she was anxious to get home quickly to look after her husband
    D. Complications may arise if she spends a long period in bed, and a long stay in hospital would result in her becoming dependent on others.

18. Nurse Davies' programme of care for Mrs Dyke while she is on traction should include:
    A. Changing her position in bed two hourly, encouraging her to drink lots of fluid and offering her bedpans frequently
    B. Massaging her buttocks two hourly with soap and water, changing her position in bed two hourly and encouraging her to drink lots of fluid
    C. Feeding her at mealtimes, massaging her buttocks two hourly with soap and water, and changing her position in bed two hourly
    D. Encouraging her to drink lots of fluid, offering her frequent bedpans and feeding her at mealtimes.

19. When Nurse Davies brought Mrs Dyke a bedpan she refused it, but a short time later she said she wanted to get up to go to the toilet. Which one of the following remarks by Nurse Davies would be most reassuring to Mrs Dyke?
    A. 'You must not get out of bed because your leg is tied'
    B. 'You cannot get up to go to the toilet so I'll give you a bedpan instead'
    C. 'You must not get out of bed because your leg is broken. Nurse and I will lift you onto this bedpan'
    D. 'I'm afraid you will have to use a bedpan. Don't worry if you make a mess — we'll soon clear it up.'

20. When cleaning Mrs Dyke after a bedpan or washing her sacral area, which one of the following statements is true?
    A. She must be lifted clear of the bed and the procedure carried out without turning her
    B. She should not be turned on to her right side because of the risk of a nerve becoming trapped between the fractured pieces of bone
    C. She should not be turned on her left side because of the risk of displacing the fracture
    D. She could be turned gently onto either side.

By the afternoon Mrs Dyke had settled quite well on the ward and she told Nurse Davies that her leg felt much more comfortable since the traction had been applied. 'It really only hurts when I move,' she said.

Despite this, she was still very anxious about her husband. At tea-time Mary arrived and Mrs Dyke was very relieved to hear that Mr Dyke had been admitted to the geriatric ward of the same hospital. While Mary was still there the medical social worker called to see Mrs Dyke.

---

21. The most likely reason for the medical social worker's call would be to:
    A. Tell Mrs Dyke that her husband had been admitted to the geriatric ward
    B. Get a full picture of Mrs Dyke's situation
    C. Collect Mrs Dyke's pension book
    D. Talk to Mary about her parent-in-law.

22. With regard to Mr and Mrs Dyke's Department of Health and Social Security pension, which one of the following statements would apply during the time they are in hospital?
    A. They will not be allowed any of their pension
    B. Their pension will be unaltered
    C. Their pension will probably be reduced when they have been in hospital for eight weeks
    D. Their pension will be reduced by half after four weeks in hospital.

The next day a nurse from the geriatric unit brought Mr Dyke in a wheelchair to see his wife. They were both delighted to see each other and Mr Dyke said he would try to visit her whenever he could. After seeing her husband Mrs Dyke was obviously very much happier and more settled.

Three days after admission Mrs Dyke was taken to the theatre for internal fixation of her sub-capital fracture.

---

23. The reason why the surgeon waited three days before operating on Mrs Dyke was to:
    A. Give her time to settle on the ward
    B. Allow her general condition to improve
    C. Enable investigations to be carried out
    D. Allow callus formation to begin.

24. Which one of the following methods of internal fixation is Mrs Dyke likely to have for the sub-capital fracture of her femur?
    A. Charnley prosthesis
    B. Smith-Petersen pin and plate
    C. Austin Moore prosthesis
    D. Küntscher nail.

25. Which one of the following would be the most likely method of nursing Mrs Dyke after her operation?
    A. On Hamilton Russell traction
    B. On simple weight and pulley traction to the right leg
    C. In a plaster of Paris hip spica
    D. Free in bed in the semi-recumbent position.

26. During the first night after her operation Mrs Dyke became mentally confused and tried to get out of bed after she had been incontinent. Having first changed her bed linen, which one of the following would be the best way for the night nurse to deal with this?
    A. Try to reassure her and offer her a bedpan frequently
    B. Give her some post-operative analgesia and make her comfortable
    C. Put sides on her bed
    D. Give her a bell and tell her to ring it if she needs a bedpan again.

The following morning when Nurse Davies came on duty, Mrs Dyke's mental and physical condition was much improved. When the surgeon did his ward round later that day he told Mrs Dyke that she would be able to sit in a chair the next morning. Three days later the physiotherapist began to teach her to walk and a week after the operation she began occupational therapy.

True/false statements *(Answers to Q. 27–31 appear on p. 139)*
The following questions (27–31) are true/false statements.

27. When getting Mrs Dyke out of bed into a chair for the first time Nurse Davies should ask a second nurse to lift her legs while she takes her shoulders and they both lift her into the chair.

28. When she is sitting in a chair both of Mrs Dyke's feet should be placed on a foot stool.

29. After this type of surgery there is less risk of deep venous thrombosis and hypostatic pneumonia if the patient sits out in a chair for the day.

30. The best way for the physiotherapist to teach Mrs Dyke to walk is with the aid of elbow crutches.

31. Mrs Dyke is likely to feel better if she gets dressed in her own clothes when she is up.

Mrs Dyke progressed well with her physiotherapy and by the time her sutures were removed she was able to walk around the ward without supervision. Mr Dyke had also received a course of physiotherapy and occupational therapy and had become much more independent.

The geriatrician and medical social worker visited Mrs Dyke and it was decided that she and her husband should have their names put on the waiting list for sheltered housing. Mrs Dyke appeared relieved by this decision as she had been worrying about how they were going to manage at home.

Multiple choice questions *(Answers to Q. 32–34 appear on pp. 139–140)*
The following questions (32–34) are multiple choice questions.

32. Sheltered housing for the elderly consists of a:
    A. Hostel with nursing staff to care for minor illnesses
    B. Flat or bungalow built especially for the elderly
    C. Flat or bungalow with a resident warden to help in emergencies
    D. Ward where elderly people get full nursing care.

33. At the occupational therapy department, Mrs Dyke would most probably participate in one of the following tasks:
    A. Use treadle sewing machine to strengthen her leg
    B. Practise dressing and coping with the toilet
    C. Knit with other elderly ladies to prevent boredom
    D. Join other patients for 'sing songs' and exercises.

34. One morning when Mrs Dyke was getting up she asked Nurse Davies to help her dress. Nurse Davies' best response would be:
    A. 'I'll stay with you and if you find anything very difficult I'll help you'
    B. 'Sister says you've got to dress yourself. If I get your clothes out you should be able to manage then'
    C. 'The occupational therapist will be along shortly to help you dress'
    D. 'Yes, of course. I'll get your clothes out and help you put them on'.

About ten weeks after she was admitted Mrs Dyke heard that a place had become available for her and Mr Dyke at Meadow Grange, which was only a few streets away from where her son lived. Mrs Dyke became quite excited when Mrs Deakin from the Social Services Department came to tell her all about her accommodation.

A very happy Mr and Mrs Dyke were collected by ambulance and taken to their new home. The medical social worker had arranged for a home help to call three mornings a week to help with housework and shopping, and a community nurse would call daily to get Mr Dyke up. Mary and her husband would call each evening to put him back to bed.

True/false statements *(Answers to Q. 35–37 appear on p. 140)*
The following questions (35–37) are true/false statements.

35. The function of the home help is to do all the housework for an elderly person.

36. The home help is not allowed to cook meals as part of her duties.

37. Mr and Mrs Dyke are likely to be charged a small fee for the home help's services.

Fractured neck of femur answers

1. **B** Of the options given, the first thing the nurse should do is to cover Mrs Dyke with a coat or blanket so that she does not become cold. Care should be taken not to overheat her as this could increase the shock. A cushion could be placed under her head so that she is more comfortable and an ambulance should be sent for (A). If it is necessary to move Mrs Dyke before the ambulance arrives, some form of splintage should be applied to prevent movement at the fracture site.

2. **D** A person who is suffering from shock has a rapid, thin pulse, the blood pressure is lowered and the face and extremities are cold and pale. In severe shock there may be signs of cyanosis present and cerebral anoxia may cause restlessness and irritability.

3. **C** The fear and pain that Mrs Dyke experienced from the fracture would cause neurogenic shock. In this type of shock the blood is shunted away from the vital organs, the surface of the body and limbs, and pools in the splanchnic (abdominal) vessels. The term 'neurogenic shock' is used to describe this type of shock because impulses pass along the vagus nerve to the blood vessels (it is sometimes referred to as vaso-vagal shock.)

   Oligaemic shock (A) is caused by a sudden severe blood loss. It is unlikely that the haemorrhage from Mrs Dyke's fracture would be severe enough to cause this type of shock.

   Toxigenic shock (B) occurs when a large quantity of toxins from damaged tissues enter the circulation and cause fluid to seep from the circulation over a large area (e.g. as in severe burns).

   Anaphylactic shock (D) is a particular type of sudden collapse which sometimes follows an injection of serum or certain drugs to which the patient is sensitive.

   (See answers 9, 10, 11 on fractured shaft of femur for further detail on shock.)

4. **A** Having already made her comfortable and prevented her from getting cold by covering her with a blanket (Question 1), the nurse should now sit beside Mrs Dyke and talk to her. A person who is afraid is usually reassured by an explanation of what is likely to happen, and the nurse holding her hand would give her additional security.

It is unwise to give her a cup of tea as a first aid measure as an anaesthetic may be required when Mrs Dyke reaches hospital (B), but Mr Dyke would be very worried about his wife and would probably appreciate a cup with a few words of reassurance. Mrs Dyke's feet should not be raised on pillows as a fracture is suspected (C), and giving her whisky to drink would increase the shock.

5. **True** Fractures of the neck of the femur are common in the elderly and occur more frequently in women then in men. This is because women live longer than men (women at 65 years have a life expectancy of 16.1 years and men at 65 of 12.2 years) and elderly women have a higher incidence of osteoporosis.

6. **True** Osteoporosis is common in the elderly, especially in women. It causes the bones to be very brittle due to lack of calcium, and frequently a trivial fall such as Mrs Dyke's can result in a fracture.

A pathological fracture caused by a secondary deposit may follow a similar minor accident, and this possibility would be eliminated by the results of X-rays.

7. **False** Fractures of the neck of the femur are classified into two groups. They are:
(a) Sub-capital fractures which lie within the capsule (inter-capsular)
(b) Trochanteric fractures which lie outside the capsule (extra-capsular).

8. **False** In an inter-trochanteric fracture the blood supply to the head of the femur remains intact, but in a sub-capital fracture the main blood vessels to the head are frequently damaged. As a result of this the main blood supply to the head of the femur would be cut off (there would still be a small amount which enters through the ligamentum teres) and avascular necrosis would occur.

The main blood vessels supplying the head of the femur run under the retinacular fibres of the capsule as it is reflected upwards along the neck before they enter the bone. They are therefore easily damaged by a sub-capital fracture.

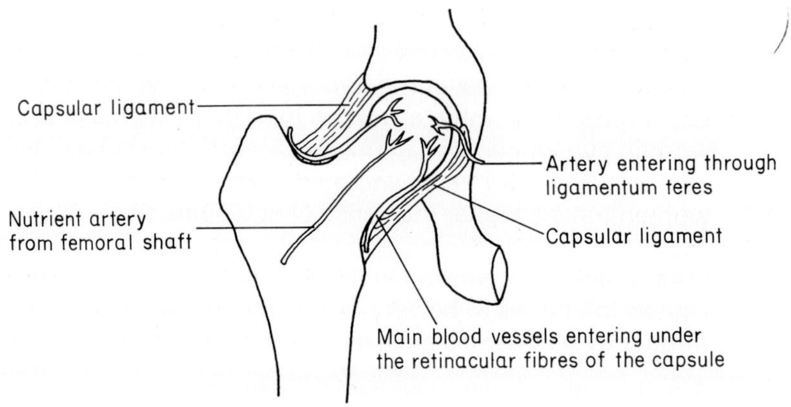

The blood supply to the head of the femur.

9. **True** About a third of sub-capital fractures do not unite despite adequate treatment (Crawford Adams, 1983). The chief reasons for this are thought to be avascular necrosis of the femoral head and incomplete immobilization.

10. **True** In addition to the two reasons given, the failure of the fracture to unite may also be due to the synovial fluid in the joint preventing the development of the initial haematoma.

11. **False** Following this type of fracture the leg is usually short and lies in lateral rotation.

12. **B** A Balkan beam attachment is necessary for the application of the Hamilton Russell traction, and a trapeze or 'monkey pole' will enable Mrs Dyke to alter her position in bed and assist the nurses with nursing procedures. Mrs Dyke will be nursed in the semi-recumbent position so a back-rest and several pillows will be required.

The bed may be of the type with a standard variable height adjustment, but this is not essential for this stage of Mrs Dyke's treatment. Because of her age and frail condition Mrs Dyke will be prone to pressure sores, so a firm mattress would not be suitable. The bed should have a soft mattress on a firm base.

13. **C** When setting up the Hamilton Russell traction, below-knee extensions are applied with a spreader at the end and a pulley (c) attached to it. A broad padded sling is placed under the knee and a cord passes from the sling over a pulley (a) which is situated on the Balkan beam distal to the knee joint. The cord then passes over pulley (b) at the foot of the bed, over pulley (c) on the spreader and finally over pulley (d) at the foot of the bed. The weight is attached to the cord and the leg placed on a pillow with the heel well clear of the mattress. The foot of the bed is elevated to provide counter-traction. (See Answer to Question 15.)

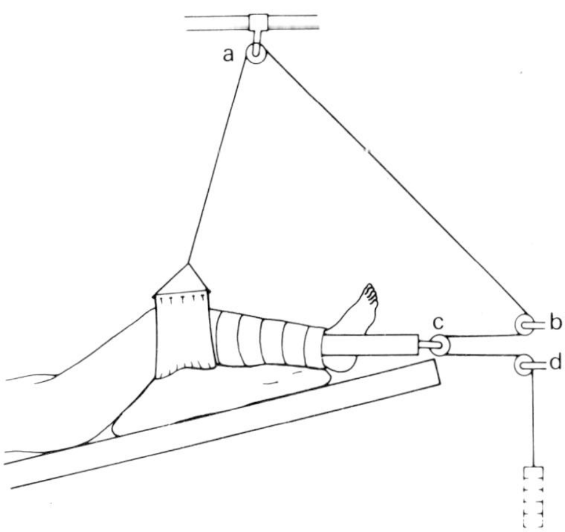

Hamilton Russell traction.

14. **A** As Mrs Dyke is likely to remain on traction for only a few days the most suitable method of applying it would be with ready-made sideways-stretch strapping extensions. Before these are put on Nurse Davies should check that there is no damage to the skin or ulcers of the lower leg. She should also make sure that Mrs Dyke is not allergic to the strapping.

Foam-backed non-adhesive extensions (B) could be used if the strapping ones were not suitable, but they tend to slip and would need to be checked often and re-applied as necessary. This type would be suitable if Mrs Dyke was going to theatre within 48 hours of admission.

As Mrs Dyke is going for surgery she is unlikely to have skeletal traction applied (C and D).

15. **B** In order that a pull can be exerted on a limb there must be two forces working in opposite directions. These forces are called traction and counter-traction. They can be applied continuously either by fixed or balanced traction.

Fixed traction (A) is exerted between two fixed points e.g. Thomas' bed knee splint. In this type of traction, the traction force is supplied by the pull of the extension tapes tied to the end of the splint and the counter-traction is the pressure of the ring of the splint on the ischial tuberosity.

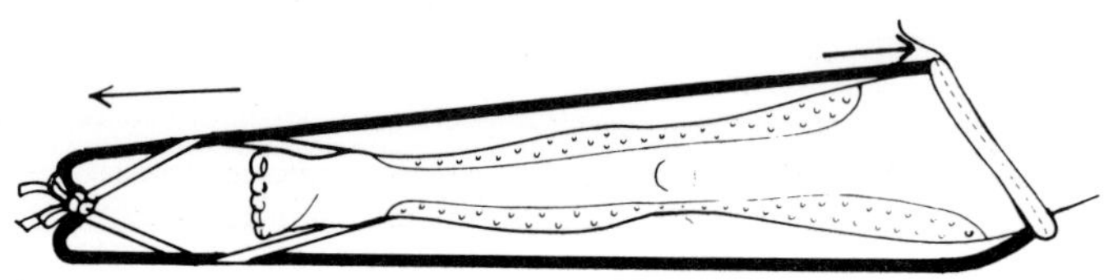

Fixed traction on a Thomas' splint.

In balanced or sliding traction, the traction force is supplied by a weight. The weight is attached to skin extensions or to a skeletal pin by a cord which runs over a pulley. Here, the counter-traction is the weight of the patient's body lying on a bed with the foot elevated, e.g. Hamilton Russell traction.

Manual traction (C) is traction which is applied by hand, e.g. when a doctor reduces a fracture; and intermittent traction (D) is applied for periods of time, e.g. in the treatment of cervical or lumbar pain.

16. C As Mrs Dyke is small and rather frail 3.5 kg weight would be adequate on the traction. A heavier person would probably require 4 kg.

The system of pulleys at the foot of the bed theoretically doubles the pull on the limb but, in practice, the friction which occurs in the system reduces this. If a parallelogram of the forces involved is drawn, it can be demonstrated that the resulting force actually pulls along the line of the femur.

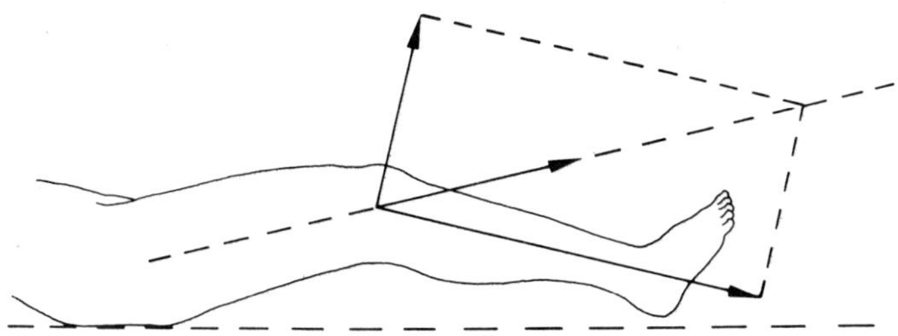

The force exerted along the line of the femur.

17. D The chief reason for early operation is that there are considerable risks of serious complications occurring if a person of Mrs Dyke's age remains in bed for a long period. Complications which could develop include pressure sores, hypostatic pneumonia and contractures of the joints. In addition, the longer she remains in hospital the more dependent she will become on other people.

Mrs Dyke would probably be very anxious to get home so that she can look after her husband, but this in itself is not a reason for performing the operation on her hip. Her fracture might unite if she was treated conservatively on Hamilton Russell traction, but the long period of bed-rest which it would entail could kill her. In addition, the possibility of avascular necrosis of the head of femur developing further increases the need to operate.

18. **A** Nurse Davies' programme of care for Mrs Dyke should centre around preventing the development of pressure sores. Areas which are especially vulnerable are the sacrum, buttocks and heels (particularly the left one which is not on traction). Mrs Dyke's position in bed should be changed every two hours and areas prone to soreness examined carefully. If her skin is soiled or damp with perspiration it should be gently washed and carefully dried, but regular massaging with soap and water could be harmful. The bottom sheet should be pulled taut, wrinkles and crumbs removed and any soiled linen replaced. Friction on the sacrum will occur if Mrs Dyke slips down the bed, so a footboard or sandbag should be placed to support her left (uninjured) foot. Should any soreness develop, aids such as a sheepskin or a ripple mattress should be used to prevent further deterioration.

Extra fluids should be given, and these are more likely to be taken if Nurse Davies finds out what drinks Mrs Dyke enjoys. Mrs Dyke will realise that if she drinks a lot she is going to need a bedpan often, so Nurse Davies should offer her a bedpan each time she is changing her position in bed. This will also help prevent incontinence.

Whenever Nurse Davies is carrying out these procedures she should encourage Mrs Dyke to lift herself up with her trapeze or 'monkey pole' and use her left leg to help. This will serve to exercise her arms and her uninjured leg. In addition, Nurse Davies should encourage her to breathe deeply, cough up any sputum and to vigorously exercise her feet to prevent deep vein thrombosis.

Mrs Dyke will probably find it difficult to do things for herself in bed but Nurse Davies should resist the temptation to do everything for her. Feeding herself might be difficult for Mrs Dyke, but the food should be cut up and the tray placed in a position where she can manage on her own. Nurse Davies should give maximum encouragement and only if it is absolutely necessary should she be fed. Similarly, Mrs Dyke should be encouraged to wash her own hands and face and brush her own teeth.

19. **C** Mrs Dyke should be told clearly why she should not get out of bed, and be reassured that the nurses will be very gentle with her when they lift her on to the bedpan. She would probably be upset if she thought the nurses expected her to make a mess of the bed (D), and correct positioning of the bedpan should prevent this.

Remarks (A) and (B) are both technically correct but are not very reassuring.

20. **D** Mrs Dyke could be turned gently on to either side without causing damage to the fracture. Movement is likely to cause pain so she will need a lot of reassurance, and the nurses should help her as much as possible, supporting her with their hands and arms. Whenever she is being lifted or moved in bed it is important that she is lifted well clear of the mattress to prevent friction on her buttocks and sacral area.

There are no important nerves closely related to the area of the femur which could become trapped (B), and a little movement of the fracture would not be detrimental, especially as it is going to be treated surgically within a few days.

21. **B** The first priority of the medical social worker is to assess the general situation so that plans can be made for both Mr and Mrs Dyke's future. The Department of Health and Social Security should be informed of Mrs Dyke's admission but it is not essential that her pension book be handed in on the first day she is admitted.

22. **C** The Department of Health and Social Security pension is not usually reduced until a patient has been in hospital for eight weeks.

23. **B** The primary reason for a few days delay before surgery is to allow an elderly person's general condition to improve. Blood and urine investigations can be carried out, chest X-rays taken and any abnormalities corrected before the operation. (In an emergency these investigations could be done very quickly and are therefore not a reason for delaying surgery.)

Providing the nursing care is of a high standard Mrs Dyke would benefit from a few days 'settling in' on the ward before her operation, and during this time minor ailments which commonly affect the elderly, such as anaemia or chest or urine infections, can be treated.

24. C Because of the risk of avascular necrosis of the head of the femur due to damage to the blood supply in a sub-capital fracture, Mrs Dyke is most likely to have the head of her femur excised and an Austin Moore or Thomson prosthesis inserted.

A Charnley prosthesis (A) is a total hip prosthesis which is generally used in arthritic conditions of the hip joint, e.g. osteoarthritis, rheumatoid arthritis or ankylosing spondylitis. (See section on osteoarthritis.)

A Smith-Petersen pin and plate (B) is one of the methods of internally fixing an inter-trochanteric fracture of the femur, and a Küntscher nail (D) is used to internally fix a fracture of the shaft of the femur.

25. D If there are no complications during the operation Mrs Dyke should not require any form of splintage or traction post-operatively. She should be nursed in the semi-recumbent position, and frequent and regular attention to her pressure areas should be continued as before her operation.

26. A It would appear that Mrs Dyke's confusion and restlessness was associated with her need to pass urine, so the night nurse should offer her a bedpan frequently during the night. Her bed should be changed and the fact that it is wet should be dealt with kindly and without chastisement. Great care should be taken to reassure her and to explain to her that she should not attempt to get out of bed but must call the nurse if she needs anything.

Efforts should be made to find out if there are any other causes for her restlessness. She may have pain and if so analgesia could be given (B), although the drugs given during the anaesthetic and the post-operative analgesic drugs may in fact be contributing to her mental confusion.

She should be watched carefully and if it is considered necessary for her own safety, bed sides (C) should be used, although these sometimes increase an elderly person's distress and nervous agitation.

Mrs Dyke could be given a bell (D), but if she is confused the nurse should not rely on her ringing it when she wants a bedpan. This should be offered to her each time observations are being taken, and whenever she is being turned or other nursing procedures are being carried out.

27. **False** It should not be necessary to lift Mrs Dyke into the chair unless the surgeon requests this. With the help of another nurse Mrs Dyke should be helped into a sitting position over the side of the bed and then, with most of her weight on her left leg, helped to stand by the bed and lowered into the chair. As with all procedures, a full explanation should be given to Mrs Dyke at the beginning and reassurance and encouragement given while she is being moved into the chair.

28. **True** Both Mrs Dyke's feet should be elevated on a foot stool in order to assist the venous return to the heart. This will prevent the pooling of blood in the deep veins of the calves and reduce the risk of deep vein thrombosis. In addition, Mrs Dyke should be encouraged to vigorously plantarflex and dorsiflex her feet.

29. **False** Sitting in a chair all day is as harmful as lying in bed with respect to these post-operative complications — and not as comfortable. Mrs Dyke should sit in a chair for about half an hour on the first day and this time should be increased as she can tolerate it. She should never be allowed to sit all day but, as her condition improves, she should be taken for short walks.

30. **False** Elbow crutches are quite difficult for old people to manage. It is much more likely that the physiotherapist would teach Mrs Dyke to walk with a walking frame.

31. **True** Getting dressed in her own clothes is likely to be a great psychological boost for Mrs Dyke once she has got over the operation. Wearing shoes is much safer than wearing slippers and makes walking easier. When she needs to rest during the day she could lie on top of the bedclothes with a blanket over her.

32. **C** Sheltered housing for the elderly generally consists of purpose-built flats or bungalows with a resident warden who can be summoned in an emergency. These may be provided by the local housing authority, housing trusts or voluntary bodies. Facilities often include a communal room for the mid-day meal and recreation, a television room and a wash room.

33. **B** The time spent in the occupational therapy department would be spent preparing for her discharge from the hospital. All activities of daily living, such as dressing, getting on and off the toilet and bed, and light housework, would be practised. Any aids for the disabled which are found to be helpful could be provided.

Mr Dyke would undergo a similar course of treatment so that he would be as independent as possible once discharged.

34. **A** In order that Mrs Dyke learns to dress herself before going home, Nurse Davies should spend the time encouraging her and only giving minimal assistance if it is required. If she finds that Mrs Dyke is having a lot of difficulty with this task, Nurse Davies should point this out to the occupational therapist so that further instruction can be given or aids provided.

35. **False** The home help should do the heavier tasks in the house, which Mr and Mrs Dyke find difficult. These would include cleaning windows, clearing out rooms and shopping. Mrs Dyke should be encouraged to do lighter tasks, like dusting, herself, so that she keeps active.

36. **False** The home help can cook a meal as part of her duties, but it is likely that Mr and Mrs Dyke would have their mid-day meal provided in the central dining room.

37. **True** A charge is made for the home help service according to the means of the elderly person. Someone who is living entirely on an 'old age pension' would have the service provided free of charge.

Meniscectomy

David Spicer is a 22-year-old car mechanic who is very keen on sport, especially football. Most Saturdays during the winter season he plays for his local football team.

During a match last October David was involved in a hard tackle with an opponent and twisted his knee, falling heavily to the ground. He complained of severe pain on the inner side of the knee and was not able to straighten it. He was carried off the field and spent the rest of the game watching on the sideline. By the end of the match his knee was swollen and he still had a lot of pain, but he was able to bend it.

He was taken to the accident and emergency department of his local hospital where his knee was examined and X-rays were taken. A provisional diagnosis of torn right medial meniscus was made.

True/false statements *(Answers to Q. 1–19 appear on pp. 147–151)*
The following questions (1–13) are true/false statements on the anatomy of the knee joint and injury to the menisci.

1. The only movements which occur at the knee joint are flexion and extension.
2. The menisci help stabilize the knee by preventing lateral displacement.
3. The cruciate ligaments are intra-capsular.
4. The tibial and fibular collateral ligaments lie within the capsule.
5. The menisci are covered with synovial membrane.
6. Tearing of the meniscus occurs when the knee is flexed and the tibia is forcibly rotated on the femur.
7. This injury is commonly seen in miners.

8. The lateral meniscus is torn more often than the medial.
9. 'Locking' of the knee in semi-flexion is a common clinical feature of a torn medial meniscus.
10. When the knee has 'locked' it cannot be flexed or extended.
11. X-Rays of the knee would show a tear in the meniscus.
12. A 'bucket handle' tear of the meniscus is one where there is a central slit with both ends attached.
13. During the examination the surgeon listened carefully while rotating the knee in flexion. He was listening for fluid splashing in the joint.

A Jones' pressure bandage was applied to David's leg. He was taught straight leg raising exercises and the nurse emphasized how important it was for him to practise these frequently throughout the day when he was at home. He was given axillary crutches and when he was able to use them with confidence he was allowed home.

David was given an appointment to attend the out-patient's department in one week.

The following questions (14–19) are true/false statements on the application of a Jones' pressure bandage.

---

14. A Jones' pressure bandage has a layer of wool applied between each layer of bandage.
15. It is applied with the knee in 10° of flexion.
16. This type of bandage should prevent knee flexion.
17. Any swelling of the knee should be controlled if the bandage is correctly applied.

18. To check the tightness of the bandage the nurse should insert two fingers between the bandage and David's leg.

19. David should be told to keep his right leg up on a footstool when he is not walking about.

Multiple choice questions *(Answers to Q. 20–33 appear on pp. 151–154)*
The remaining questions in this case history are multiple choice questions.

---

20. Swelling of a joint is:
    A. Haemarthrosis
    B. Effusion
    C. Haematoma
    D. Oedema.

21. Straight leg raising exercises are carried out to strengthen the:
    A. Hamstring muscles
    B. Psoas muscle
    C. Quadriceps muscle
    D. Gluteal muscle.

22. When selecting crutches for David the nurse should make sure that his weight is taken on his hands to avoid damaging the:
    A. Axillary nerve
    B. Radial nerve
    C. Axillary artery
    D. Brachial artery.

When David visited the out-patient's department a week later his knee had improved considerably and the surgeon advised a course of physiotherapy. However, after a few weeks of this treatment it became apparent that he still had considerable problems with the joint.

The surgeon told him that he thought he would need to have the damaged meniscus removed, and early in the new year he was admitted for an arthroscopy and probable meniscectomy. The arthroscopy showed that David had a 'bucket handle' tear of the right medial meniscus and a meniscectomy was performed.

23. An arthroscopy is:
    A. An examination of a joint using special heat-detecting equipment
    B. An X-ray of a joint following an injection of radio-opaque fluid
    C. A surgical exploration of a joint
    D. An examination of the internal structures of a joint with a special telescopic instrument.

24. A meniscectomy was not performed when David first injured his knee because:
    A. It is unwise to operate when there is swelling of the joint
    B. The surgeon hoped the tear would repair itself
    C. He was in a shocked condition after the accident
    D. The surgeon was not certain of the diagnosis.

25. When operating on David the surgeon found that the peripheral portion of the meniscus was attached to the bone so he would most likely remove:
    A. Both menisci in that knee
    B. The part of the meniscus which had become detached
    C. The whole of the meniscus which is damaged
    D. The damaged meniscus and replace it with a sylastic implant.

26. Following his meniscectomy David's knee would most likely be immobilized:
    A. On a Thomas' splint with skin traction
    B. On a metal gutter splint with the knee at 10° of flexion
    C. In a crêpe bandage
    D. In a Jones' pressure bandage.

27. After recovering from the anaesthetic David should be instructed to:
    A. Do straight leg raising exercises for 5 minutes in every hour
    B. Rest the leg so that it does not become too painful
    C. Begin gentle knee flexion as his pain allows
    D. Try to lift his leg up straight when he thinks he can manage it.

28. The post-operative analgesia prescribed was pethidine 100 mg to be given 4 to 6 hourly as required. The nurse should:
    A. Only give it if David's pain becomes very severe
    B. Withhold it for the first 24 hours so that he will be able to do his exercises
    C. Give it regularly every 4 to 6 hours
    D. Give it whenever he complains of pain.

Three days after the operation David's dressing was reduced and a light supporting bandage was applied to his knee. The surgeon allowed him out of bed with crutches and ordered knee flexion exercises and more intensive physiotherapy.

---

29. When teaching David to walk with crutches the physiotherapist should instruct him to:
    A. Take no weight on the affected leg
    B. Take a little weight on the affected leg and keep his knee straight when weightbearing
    C. Take a little weight on the affected leg and flex his knee as much as the pain will allow
    D. Walk normally but use his crutches if he needs extra support.

30. More intensive quadriceps exercises are achieved by:
    A. Lying the patient prone and instructing him to extend his hip
    B. Lying the patient supine and instructing him to lift his leg up straight
    C. Instructing the patient to lift his leg up straight with his legs abducted
    D. Applying weights to the foot and instructing the patient to lift his leg up straight.

31. When David is being taught his knee-flexion exercises he should be:
    A. Lying on the bed and gently flexing the knee within the limits of pain
    B. Lying on the bed and forcing the knee into flexion
    C. Sitting on the side of the bed and swinging the leg
    D. Sitting on the side of the bed with a weight attached to the foot and allowing the leg to swing.

David progressed well with his physiotherapy. His sutures were removed on the tenth day after the operation and two days later he was discharged home. He was to attend out-patient physiotherapy three days a week.

32. Which of the following replies is the surgeon most likely to make when David asks if he would be able to play football again?
    A. 'No, you will never be able to play again'
    B. 'No, nor will you be able to continue as a mechanic because of the strain on your knees'
    C. 'Yes, but you must wait a year before you play again'
    D. 'Yes, once your knee has recovered you will be able to play again'.

33. Which one of the following conditions is David most likely to suffer from in later life because of his injury?
    A. Osteochondritis
    B. Osteoporosis
    C. Osteoarthritis
    D. Osteomalacia.

Meniscectomy answers

1. **False** The main movements of the knee joint are flexion and extension with a small degree of rotation. When the knee is flexed it can be slightly internally and externally rotated, and with the knee fully extended a small amount of rotation occurs which 'locks' the joint into a stable position. These rotationary movements give extra strength and stability to the joint.

2. **True** The menisci are crescent-shaped discs of fibro-cartilage which are thicker on the outer edges. They are attached to the superior surface of the rather flat tibial condyles and give extra stability to the joint by forming shallow sockets for the condyles of the femur.

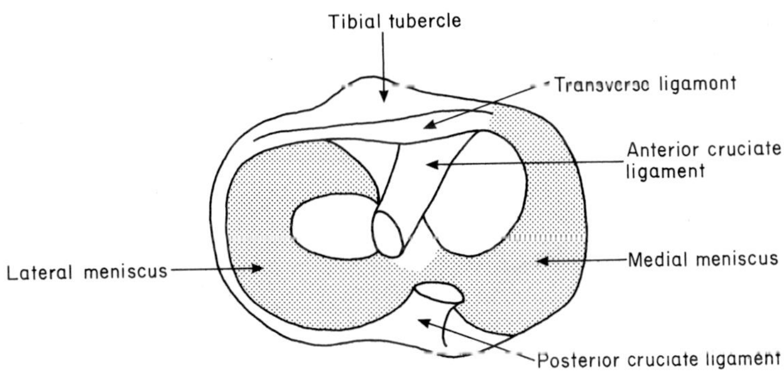

A transverse section of the knee showing the medial and lateral menisci.

3. **True** There are two cruciate ligaments extending from the inter-condylar notch of the femur to the inter-condylar eminence of the tibia. The posterior cruciate ligament has a fan-shaped proximal attachment on the anterior part of the medial femoral condyle and distally it is attached to the tibia and the posterior part of the lateral meniscus. The anterior cruciate ligament is attached proximally to the posterior part of the lateral femoral condyle and distally to the anterior part of the tibia between the condyles.

As their name suggests they cross and in this way they give stability to the joint.

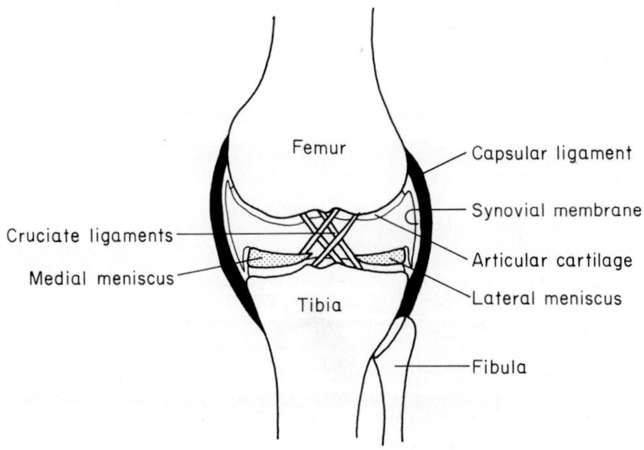

Coronal section of the knee joint showing the internal structures.

4. **False** The tibial and fibular collateral ligaments are supporting ligaments of the knee which lie outside the capsule. The tibial (medial) ligament blends with the capsule but the fibular (lateral) ligament is separate. The anterior part of the capsule is strengthened by the ligamentum patellae.

5. **False** The menisci are discs of fibro-cartilage which are not covered by synovial membrane. The above figure shows the synovial membrane lining the inner surface of the joint capsule and also covering the cruciate ligaments.

6. **True** In a young person the meniscus is only torn when the weight is being taken on the leg, the knee is flexed and the tibia is forcibly rotated on the femur. In an older person the meniscus is less mobile and may tear with little force.

7. **True** Because miners work in a crouched position they are particularly prone to this injury. In addition it is a very common injury sustained by athletes, especially footballers.

8. **False** Tears of the medial meniscus are three times more common than tears of the lateral meniscus. This is because the medial meniscus is attached to the tibial (medial) collateral ligament, whereas the lateral meniscus is more mobile.

9. **True** The joint may become 'locked' in 10–20 degrees of flexion when a torn piece of cartilage becomes jammed between the articulating surfaces. A torn lateral meniscus rarely causes 'locking' of the joint.

10. **False** Once the knee becomes 'locked', extension is not possible without a manipulation, or sometimes it 'unlocks' spontaneously. It is usually possible to fully flex the knee.

11. **False** Cartilage does not show up on X-rays. X-rays are usually taken to check that there are no loose bodies in the joint or that there are no fractures, such as a fracture of the tibial spine.

12. **True** There are three types of slits which may occur in the medial meniscus.
They are:
(a) A tear of the anterior horn
(b) A tear of the posterior horn
(c) A central slit along the length of the meniscus with the two ends still attached — a 'bucket handle' tear. The loose portion often lies in the inter-condylar notch and may cause the knee to lock.
The point at which the meniscus tears depends on the degree of flexion of the knee at the moment of injury.

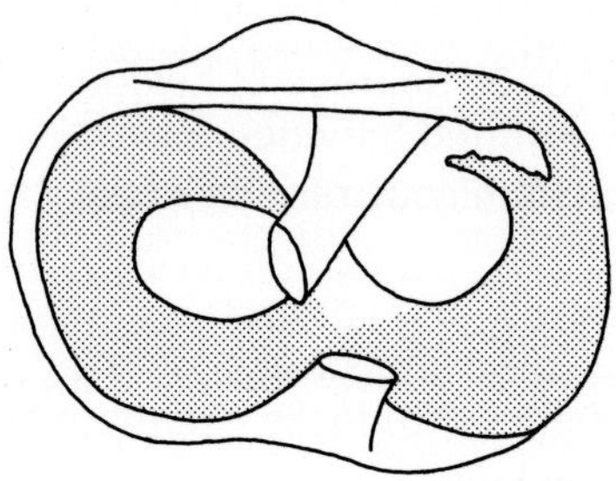

(a) a tear of the anterior horn

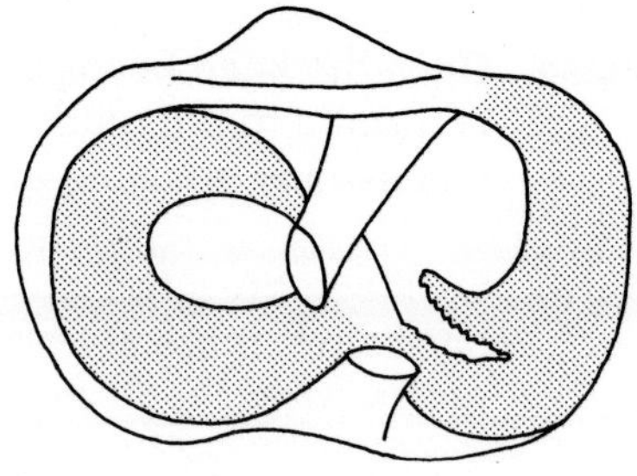

(b) a tear of the posterior horn

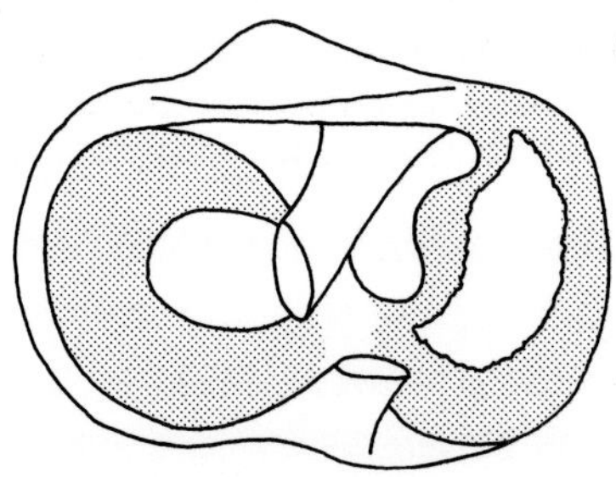

(c) a 'bucket handle' tear.

13. **False** Once the swelling of the knee has settled after the initial injury, the surgeon would carry out the McMurray's test to confirm the diagnosis. This test is done with the patient lying in the supine position and relaxed. The knee is fully flexed, externally rotated and extended in abduction. The surgeon keeps his hand over the joint line while putting the knee through these movements and, if the cartilage is torn, he may feel a click, the patient may complain of pain or the cartilage may even be felt to protrude.

    This test is not usually carried out when the knee is acutely painful and swollen.

14. **True** When applying a Jones' pressure bandage a layer of splint-wool is first wrapped around the knee. The bandage is then applied, starting with three firm turns around the knee; then another layer of splint-wool is added and another layer of bandage — this is continued until the whole of the bandage is used up.

15. **False** This type of bandage is applied with the knee in full extension.

16. **True** The bandage is applied tight enough to prevent any flexion of the joint.

17. **True** As well as keeping the knee in full extension the bandage should control joint swelling.

18. **False** If the bandage has been correctly applied the nurse will not be able to insert two fingers between it and David's skin. The colour, sensation and movement of his foot should be checked carefully before he leaves the hospital and he should be told to return at once if his foot should swell or if numbness or discoloration should develop.

19. **True** In order to assist the venous return and to prevent (or reduce) the swelling, David should be told to elevate his foot on a footstool when he is not walking about.

20. **B** An effusion of a joint is a collection of fluid in the joint causing it to swell. The fluid is frequently an abnormal volume of synovial fluid which has been produced in response to injury to avascular structures within the knee or to inflammator changes. In infective conditions, pus may be present, or after severe trauma there may be blood in the joint—haemarthrosis (A). As the menisci are avascular, haemarthrosis would not normally occur after they are injured. A haematoma (C) is a collection of blood in the tissues and oedema (D) is when fluid collects in the tissues.

21. **C** Active exercises of the quadriceps muscle are important after any knee injury in order to regain stability of the joint. Once the patient can lift his leg up straight with ease, weights may be attached to the foot in order to increase the resistance and further strengthen the muscle.

Strong quadriceps muscles are vital for knee stability when a person is standing and walking.

22. **B** It is important that the correct length of axillary crutches are given to David so that he takes the weight of his body on his hands rather than on his axillae. Pressure from the crutch could damage the radial nerve as it passes through the axilla, causing the injury known as 'crutch palsy'.

23. **D** An arthroscopy is an examination of the internal structures of a joint using a special telescopic instrument called an arthroscope. The procedure is carried out under a general anaesthetic and the internal structures of the joint are examined with a fibre-optic viewer. A recent advance has been to perform a 'closed meniscectomy' through the arthroscope, i.e. the torn part of the meniscus is removed. This is a rather difficult procedure but when it is carried out successfully the recovery is rapid.

The use of a heat-detecting instrument for examining areas of the body is called thermography (A), and a surgical exploration of a joint is an arthrotomy (C). X-raying a joint after injecting radio-opaque fluid or air into it is an arthrogram (B) and this may be used to confirm the diagnosis of a torn meniscus.

24. **A** A meniscectomy should not be performed until the effusion of the knee has resolved. The menisci do not have a blood supply, so healing of the tear will not take place (B), although partial regeneration does sometimes occur after the meniscus has been removed.

The injury is frequently very painful but the degree of shock is not usually severe so this would not be a contra-indication for surgery (C). There may be some doubt about the diagnosis (D), which would only be confirmed by an arthrogram or an arthroscopy, neither of which should be carried out while the knee is very swollen.

25. **B** When the peripheral portion of the torn meniscus is found to be intact it is usual to remove the loose fragment and leave the attached portion in place. If the peripheral attachment is damaged, the whole of the damaged cartilage would then be removed (C).
N.B. Some surgeons remove the whole meniscus even when the peripheral attachment is undamaged.

There is no point in removing both menisci as the joint will function better with one than with none at all (A). At the present time artificial replacement of the cartilage is not carried out (D).

26. **D** Each surgeon has his own method of immobilizing the knee following a meniscectomy. Probably the most common method used is a pressure bandage to control the swelling and to keep the knee in full extension. A metal or other type of gutter splint may be incorporated but the knee should always be fully extended (never at 10° of flexion (B)). Occasionally a plaster of Paris cylinder may be used or plaster of Paris over a pressure bandage.

A crêpe bandage alone (C) would not control the swelling or movement sufficiently and a Thomas' splint with skin traction (A) would not allow the patient to mobilize or carry out his exercises.

27. **A** Straight leg raising exercises should have been taught before the operation and should begin as soon as David is sufficiently recovered from the anaesthetic. The nursing staff should give encouragement and supervise these exercises when the physiotherapist is not available, and they should be practised for 5 minutes in every hour during the day.

28. **C** During the first 24 hours after the operation the analgesia should be given regularly and not just when David complains of pain. This means that the pain will be kept at a constant low level and he will be able to practise his exercises with the minimum of discomfort.

29. **B** When David starts walking with crutches he is allowed to take some weight on the affected leg, but his knee must be fully extended when the weight is being transmitted through that knee.

30. **D** Weight added to the foot during straight leg raising exercises increases the effort required to lift the foot up, and consequently the strength of the quadriceps muscle. The weight is increased as the muscle strength develops.

31. **A** Knee-flexion exercises should be very gentle at first and within the limits of pain. This is best achieved with the patient lying on the bed so that his leg is fully supported. Forcibly flexing the knee (B), sitting over the side of the bed and using a swinging action (C) or a weight (D) to increase the knee flexion are all dangerous and could cause damage to the supporting structures of the joint.

32. **D** There is no reason why David should not play football again once his knee has recovered, but the time this will take will depend largely on how quickly he recovers and develops the muscle control of the joint. This will mean a lot of hard work for David.

33. **C** Probably the commonest cause of post-traumatic osteoarthritis of the knee joint in middle-aged and elderly men is damage to the menisci. As well as giving stability to the joint the menisci act as shock absorbers within the joint, so if they are damaged, or removed, there will be an increase in the amount of stress on the articulating cartilages which could be the cause of osteoarthritis of the knee.

Colles' fracture

Mrs Freda Southall is a 65-year-old housewife who tripped while hanging out the washing in the garden and fell on to her outstretched left hand. Her husband took her to the family doctor at once as she was complaining of severe pain in her wrist. The doctor examined the wrist and sent her to the accident and emergency department of the local hospital as he suspected that the wrist was fractured. X-rays taken on arrival confirmed that she had a left Colles' fracture with the classic 'dinner fork' deformity.

Multiple choice questions *(Answers to Q. 1–3 appear on pp. 160)*
Questions 1–3 are multiple choice type questions.

1. A Colles' fracture is:
   A. An oblique fracture of the lower ulna
   B. A fracture of the radius and ulna within 5 cm of the wrist joint
   C. An oblique fracture of the radius with dislocation of the wrist joint
   D. A transverse fracture of the lower radius.

2. This type of fracture is particularly common in elderly women because of the presence of:
   A. Osteomalacia
   B. Osteoporosis
   C. Osteochondritis
   D. Osteoarthritis.

3. Which one of the following is *not* found in the classic 'dinner fork' deformity seen in this type of fracture?
   A. Impaction of the wrist
   B. Dorsal displacement of the distal fragment
   C. Volar displacement of the lower radius
   D. Lateral displacement of the lower radius.

The casualty officer explained to Mrs Southall that she would need a general anaesthetic in order to reduce the fracture. As it was over four hours since she had received anything to eat or drink she was able to have the anaesthetic at once. The fracture was reduced and the wrist immobilized in a dorsal-radial plaster of Paris slab.

Matching item questions *(Answers to Q. 4–6 appear on pp. 161–162)*
The following questions (4–6) are matching item questions about the reduction of a Colles' fracture.

From the list on the left select the appropriate description of each stage of the reduction listed on the right.

A. The distal fragment pressed in the volar direction and the wrist flexed
B. Traction applied to the hand and dorsiflexion of the distal fragment
C. Extension of the wrist and the distal fragment pressed in the dorsal direction
D. Pronation of the distal fragment and ulnar deviation
E. Supination of the distal fragment and radial deviation.

4. Disimpaction
5. Reduction
6. Locking in position.

True/false statements *(Answers to Q. 7–26 appear on pp. 162–166)*
The following questions (7–26) are true/false statements.

---

7. The dorsal-radial plaster of Paris slab should extend over the elbow joint.

8. Distally, the slab should extend over the metacarpal heads.

9. The slab should cover two thirds of the circumference of the forearm.

10. Ten minutes after applying the slab it is covered with a crêpe bandage.

Mrs Southall soon regained consciousness after the anaesthetic and the casualty officer ordered an X-ray of her arm in the plaster. He was pleased to see that the position of the fracture was satisfactory. He checked that she was comfortable in the plaster and that there was no impairment to the nerve or to the blood supply to the fingers.

Mrs Southall was allowed a period of rest before being allowed home. She was given written instructions about the care of her plaster and these were explained fully to her. In addition, she was taught how to exercise the joints of her left arm which were not immobilized.

Appointments were made for her to return the next day to have her plaster checked and for a weeks time for further X-rays.

---

11. Before being discharged Mrs Southall should have her arm placed in a sling which she should be instructed to wear for a full week.

12. She should be told to start exercising her shoulder and elbow immediately but she should avoid movement of her fingers for the first two days.

13. Shoulder exercises are particularly important for Mrs Southall because she fell on to her outstretched hand.

14. She should be told to use the hand as much as possible as long as she does not wet the plaster.

15. As the weather was cold Mrs Southall was told that she could use a hair dryer to dry the plaster more quickly.

16. She was instructed to remove her wedding ring if there was any sign of her fingers swelling.

17. She should be told to return to the hospital at once if her fingers begin to swell.

18. If Mrs Southall returned to the hospital with badly swollen and discoloured fingers, the correct action would be to split the bandage from the palm to the elbow.

19. If the plaster should crack she should return to the hospital.

Mrs Southall felt much better the next day but her hand was still rather painful and her fingers a little swollen. The doctor reassured her that all was well and she was again told of the importance of continuing with her exercises.

X-rays taken a week later showed the fracture to be still in a satisfactory position. All the swelling had subsided and it was decided to convert the plaster of Paris slab into a full Colles' plaster.

Mrs Southall was seen again three weeks after the injury and X-rays were taken to check the position of the fracture.

---

20. The dorsal-radial plaster of Paris slab must be converted into a full Colles' plaster within the first week of the injury.

21. It is not necessary to remove the plaster slab in order to apply a full Colles' plaster.

22. When treating a Colles' fracture the plaster is usually kept on for six weeks after the injury.

No complications occurred and when Mrs Southall had her plaster removed a crêpe bandage was applied for support. She was told to begin exercising her wrist in order to regain full movement.

When she visited the clinic for the last time six weeks later, Mrs Southall said that her wrist was still a bit weak but was getting stronger and that she was now able to do most things with her left hand. She was told that if she had any further problems she should consult her family foctor.

---

23. The best way of achieving full wrist movement is for Mrs Southall to use her hand for normal domestic tasks such as washing dishes.

24. Mal-union of a Colles' fracture is not often seen as the reduction is relatively simple and easily maintained.

25. The tendon of extensor pollicis longus may rupture when the Colles' fracture occurs.

26. Stiffness of the shoulder or fingers does not occur in a young person with this type of fracture.

Matching item questions *(Answers to Q. 27–29 appear on pp. 166–167)*
The next 3 questions (27–29) are matching item questions related to the complications of a Colles' fracture.

From the list on the left select the appropriate symptoms for each of the complications of Colles' fracture listed on the right.

A. Painful, stiff and swollen fingers and hand
B. Pain, tingling and numbness of the thumb, index and middle fingers at night
C. Severe pain on passive stretching of fingers with pale skin of the hand
D. Pain on the radial side of the wrist, particularly on rotation
E. Pain over the dorsum of the wrist and swelling over the head of the ulna.

27. Carpal tunnel compression
28. Subluxation of inferior radio-ulnar joint
29. Sudeck's atrophy.

Colles' fracture answers

1. **D** A Colles' fracture is a transverse fracture of the radius which occurs less than 2.5 cm from the wrist joint. There may be an associated fracture of the ulnar styloid.

An oblique fracture of the lower radius with dislocation of the wrist joint (C) is called a Barton's fracture.

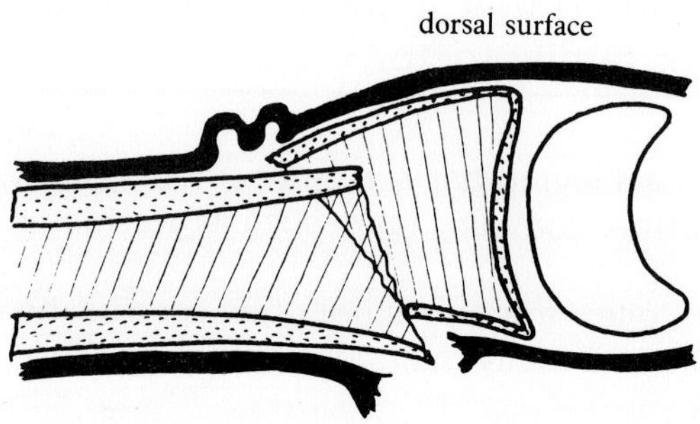

Colles' fracture.

2. **B** This type of fracture occurs most commonly in elderly women because their bones are particularly brittle due to post-menopausal osteoporosis. Frequently, the accident which causes the fracture is relatively trivial, such as stumbling and falling onto the outstretched hand.
3. **C** The classic deformity of a Colles' fracture is the 'dinner fork' deformity where there is dorsal (backward) displacement and tilting of the distal fragment (B) as well as lateral (radial) displacement (D). The fragments are commonly impacted (A).

Not all patients with a Colles' fracture demonstrate this deformity. Where the fracture is not displaced and the deformity is less obvious, the clinical features are local tenderness and pain on movement.

Volar (forward) displacement of the distal fragment (C) is seen in a Smith's fracture. This is sometimes referred to as a reverse Colles' fracture.

4. **B**
5. **A**
6. **D**

There are three stages in the reduction of a Colles' fracture — disimpaction, reduction and locking the fracture into the reduced position. During all three stages an assistant holds the elbow and provides countertraction.

Disimpaction of the fracture is achieved by the surgeon applying traction to the hand and at the same time increasing the existing backward displacement by dorsiflexing the distal fragment (B).

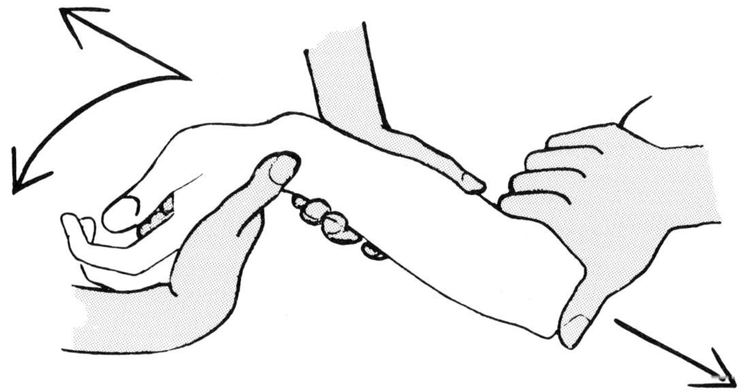

Once the fracture has been disimpacted, it can be reduced by the surgeon pressing the distal fragment in the volar direction and flexing the wrist (A). The surgeon's other hand provides counter-pressure on the proximal fragment. At the end of this stage the fracture is fully reduced but is unstable.

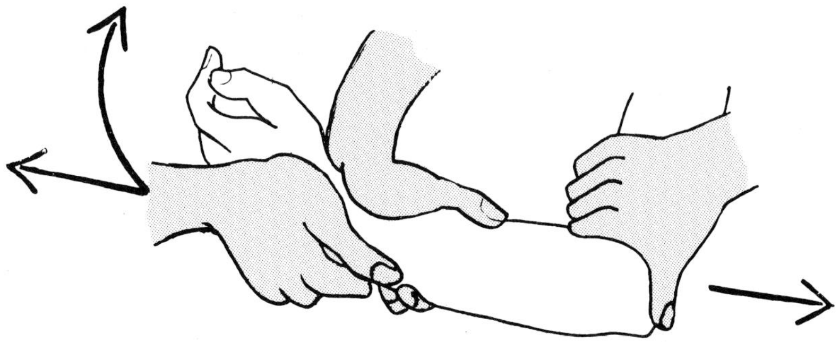

The final stage of the reduction is the locking of the fracture into a stable position. This is achieved by pronating the hand and the distal fragment and deviating the wrist to the ulna (D). The fracture is thus locked in a stable position so that the plaster can be applied.

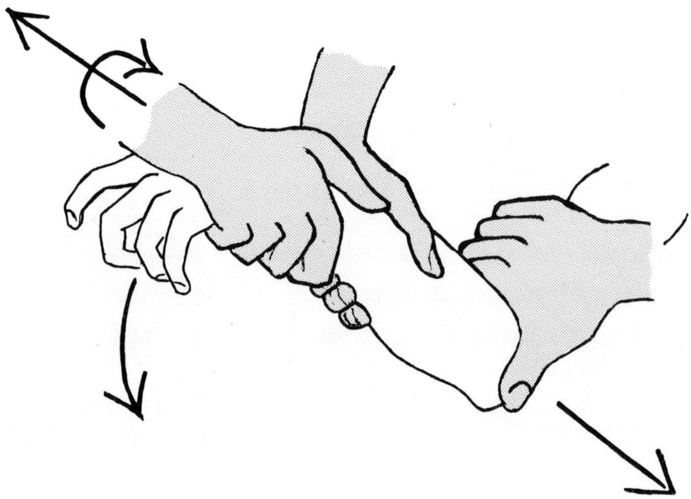

It is usually necessary to give the patient a general anaesthetic in order to carry out this reduction in a displaced Colles' fracture.

7. **False** The plaster slab usually extends to just below the elbow, allowing sufficient room for full flexion of the elbow joint to take place.

8. **False** Distally the plaster should extend no further than the distal palmar crease (or the metacarpal necks), thus allowing room for full flexion of the fingers.

9. **True** In order that the dorsal-radial plaster of Paris slab effectively holds the fracture in the reduced position, it must cover two thirds of the circumference of the forearm. It is important that the plaster is thick enough to allow firm pressure to be applied by the surgeon who holds the fracture while the plaster is setting.

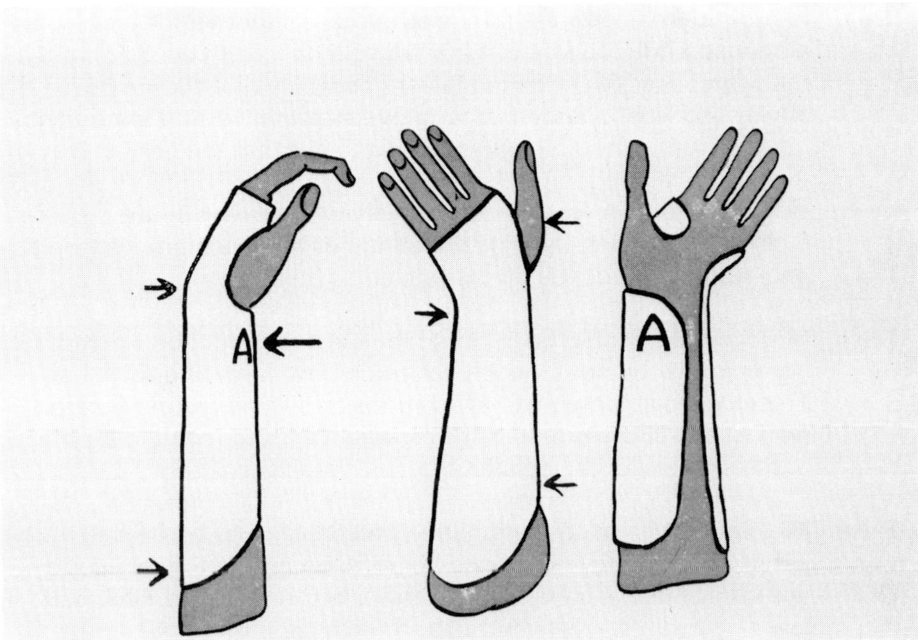

10. **False** Once the plaster slab has been moulded to the forearm it is usual to apply a wet gauze or conforming bandage to hold the slab in position.

11. **False** Mrs Southall should be told to discard the sling after the first day or two when the swelling has subsided. She should be instructed that in the mean time she should remove her arm from the sling frequently so that she can exercise her fingers, elbow and shoulder.

12. **False** Finger exercises should be carried out immediately, however painful they may be: in fact, the greater the swelling of the fingers, the greater is the importance of exercising them.

13. **True** In view of Mrs Southall's age, and the fact that her shoulder might have been slightly damaged in the fall, there is a considerable risk of a 'frozen shoulder' developing. In order to prevent this occurring, it is vital that nursing and medical staff should emphasize the importance of maintaining the movement of the shoulder while her wrist is immobilized.

14. **True** In order to maintain the movement of her shoulder, as well as her elbow and fingers, Mrs Southall should be told to use her hand as much as possible once the plaster has dried. She should be advised to wear a large rubber glove to protect it and to prevent it getting wet. It should be pointed out to her that the easiest way of exercising all the joints of her left arm which are not immobilized in the plaster is to use the hand freely when carrying out everyday activities, such as brushing her hair, cleaning her teeth, and most light household tasks such as dusting.

15. **False** Mrs Southall should be told that the plaster should be allowed to dry naturally without the application of any form of direct heat. To dry the plaster with a hair dryer or by similar means of direct heat would cause the plaster to crack and could result in burning of the skin under the plaster.

16. **False** Mrs Southall's wedding ring, and any other rings on her left hand, should have been removed as soon as she arrived in the accident and emergency department, before swelling occurs. If swelling has already occurred and the rings cannot be removed, consent should be obtained from Mrs Southall and the rings cut off.

Mrs Southall or her husband should sign a receipt for any jewellery and other items when they are handed over.

17. **False** Mrs Southall should be told that some swelling of the fingers is to be expected. If this occurs she should lie down and support her arm with pillows so that her fingers point to the ceiling. If the swelling persists and the fingers become discoloured, painful or numb, then she should be told to return to the hospital at once.

18. **True** If elevation of the arm does not succeed in reducing the swelling, the doctor should be informed and, with his permission, the bandage should be split to the skin from the palm to the elbow. A crêpe bandage should then be applied.

19. **True** Mrs Southall should be told to return to the hospital if the plaster cracks or becomes soft at any time during the period of immobilization. Failure to do so may result in the fracture slipping, causing mal-union, or pressure may develop under the plaster.

20. **False** Many surgeons treat their patients with a Colles' fracture in only a dorsal-radial slab, while others prefer not to use a slab at all and apply a complete Colles' plaster at the time of the injury. The advantage of a dorsal-radial slab is that if swelling occurs after the reduction of the fracture the bandage can be split easily without displacement of the fracture, and as the swelling subsides a firmer bandage can be applied.

    Some surgeons convert the dorsal-radial slab into a full Colles' plaster at about 7 to 10 days after the injury, when the swelling has gone down.

21. **True** The usual procedure is to split the gauze bandage and apply the plaster of Paris bandages over the plaster slab. Again, it is important to ensure that there is no restriction of elbow and metacarpophalangeal joint movement.

    If X-rays show that displacement of the fracture has occurred, it may be necessary to remove the plaster slab so that the fracture can be remanipulated before a full Colles' plaster is applied.

    Mrs Southall should be advised to wear her sling for 24 hours until the plaster is dry and then it can be discarded. The importance of exercising her fingers, elbow and shoulder should again be stressed.

22. **True** The average time it takes for a Colles' fracture to unite is five to six weeks. The plaster is then removed and a supporting bandage is applied. It must be said that at this stage the fracture is not consolidated but it is firm enough to prevent displacement occurring.

    Even if the union is not particularly good or the position of the fracture is not entirely satisfactory, it is not usually advisable to continue the splintage longer than six weeks as this will lead to joint stiffness.

23. **True** The best way of exercising her wrist is for Mrs Southall to use it when doing light housework but this should be within the limits of pain. Lifting heavy weights with her left hand should be avoided initially.

24. **False** Mal-union of a Colles' fracture is fairly common and usually occurs because reduction has not been complete or has not been maintained in the plaster. It leads to deformity with weakness and loss of rotation and is usually treated with physiotherapy.

25. **False** Rupture of the extensor pollicis longus tendon is a complication of a Colles' fracture, but the rupture usually occurs about 4 weeks after the injury or sometimes later. The reason for the rupture occurring is thought to be damage to the blood supply to the tendon during the initial injury. This leads to fraying of the tendon until finally it ruptures.

    The treatment is usually to repair the tendon by transplanting the extensor indicis tendon and attaching it to the distal stump of the extensor pollicis longus.

26. **False** Unless the shoulder and fingers are used and exercised when the plaster is in position, stiffness of the shoulder and fingers will occur, even in a young person. In an older person stiffness, should it occur, is a serious problem because regaining movement is very difficult, especially of the shoulder joint. It is therefore vital that all patients with a Colles' fracture, whatever their age, understand the importance of carrying out their exercises correctly.

27. **B** Compression of the median nerve within the carpal tunnel may be caused by persistent backward displacement of the distal fragment of the radius if a complete reduction has not been achieved and maintained. This gives rise to pain and paraesthesia in the distribution of the median nerve which characteristically occurs at night.

    If the compression is severe and the symptoms persist, decompression of the carpal tunnel is performed.

28. **E** Subluxation of the inferior radio-ulnar joint may occur if the fracture is not adequately reduced or the position is lost after reduction. This gives rise to pain over the radio-ulnar joint and impaired wrist movement, especially adduction and rotation. The head of the ulna is prominent.

In a young person the treatment is to excise the lower end of the ulna if the condition is severe and causing a lot of trouble.

29. **A** Sudeck's atrophy is a condition which is not fully understood but it occasionally follows fractures or injuries to the limbs. Colles' fracture is the commonest cause of the condition.

It occurs about two months after the injury. The hand and fingers become painful, very swollen and the skin is stretched and shiny. The joints become stiff, especially the metacarpophalangeal and interphalangeal joints, leading to a condition sometimes referred to as a 'frozen hand'.

The treatment is prolonged and intensive physiotherapy.

Fractured shaft of femur

Matthew Ingelson is 18 years old, and for several years his greatest ambition has been to own a motor cycle. Since he began working as a builder's labourer two years ago he has saved hard, and on his 18th birthday his parents made up the money so that he could buy a second-hand motor cycle.

He was delighted with it. Each evening he and his friends would ride around on their motor cycles and they spent quite a lot of time in a disused quarry just outside the town putting their bikes through their paces.

One wet night in October he was returning home at about 11.00 p.m. when a car drew out of a side street near the town centre and knocked Matthew off his motor cycle. He lay on the road with his left leg badly twisted and with severe pain in his thigh. He was fully conscious and talking normally.

A lady arrived on the scene almost at once, offering her services as a first-aider. She thought that Matthew probably had a fracture of his left femur but, other than a superficial graze on his forehead, he appeared to have no other injuries.

Multiple choice questions *(Answers to Q. 1–5 appear on pp. 175–176)*
The following questions (1–5) are multiple choice questions.

1. Having ascertained that Matthew was conscious and breathing normally which one of the following actions would have the greatest priority for the first-aider?
   A. Telephone for an ambulance
   B. Immobilize Matthew's leg
   C. Stop oncoming traffic
   D. Evaluate Matthew's injuries.

2. Which one of the following would be the best course of action in view of the fact that the only obvious injury was a fracture of the shaft of the femur?
   A. Make him comfortable and cover him with a coat
   B. Tie his feet together with a belt having corrected the deformity, and move him into a shop doorway
   C. Tie his legs to a stick or broom handle and remove his helmet
   D. Gently ease him onto the pavement and give him a drop of whisky to ease the pain.

3. As Matthew was talking normally which one of the following questions would be the most important for the first-aider to ask?
   A. 'When did you last have something to drink?'
   B. 'Have you been drinking alcohol?'
   C. 'How old are you?'
   D. 'Do you remember the accident?'

4. In accordance with the Road Traffic Act 1972, Matthew may later be asked to pay a fee for the emergency treatment because the:
   A. Accident occurred on a public road
   B. Ambulance attended in response to a 999 call
   C. Accident involved a licensed vehicle
   D. Ambulance attended after normal 9.00 a.m. to 5.00 p.m. duty hours.

5. When Matthew arrived at the accident and emergency department, which one of the following should the nurse attending him do first?
   A. Put an identification band on his arm
   B. Undress him so that the doctor can examine him
   C. Check that the resuscitation equipment is close at hand should it be needed urgently.
   D. Take and record his vital signs, pupil reactions and level of consciousness.

On his arrival at the hospital Matthew's blood pressure was 100/60 mmHg and his pulse was 130 beats per minute, indicating that he was moderately shocked. The casualty officer started an intravenous infusion of normal saline and a specimen of blood was taken for grouping and cross-matching.

X-rays taken showed that Matthew had a transverse fracture of the lower third of his left femur. A general anaesthetic was given and his leg was immobilized in a Thomas' splint with skeletal traction.

Matching item questions *(Answers to Q. 6–11 appear on pp. 177–179)*
The following two groups of questions (6–11) are of the matching items type.

6–8 From the list on the left select the blood groups which could be given to each patient in the list on the right.

A. O Rhesus negative or B Rhesus negative
B. B Rhesus positive or AB Rhesus negative
C. O Rhesus positive or A Rhesus negative
D. O Rhesus positive
E. AB Rhesus positive.

6. A patient with blood group A positive
7. A patient with blood group B negative
8. A patient with blood group O positive.

9–11 From the list on the left select the event which might lead to each type of shock listed on the right.

A. Severe blood loss following the severing of a major blood vessel
B. Collapse after standing for a long period in hot sunshine
C. Gradual seepage of fluid from the capillaries following severe burns
D. Sudden collapse following the administration of a drug.

9. Oligaemic shock
10. Neurogenic shock
11. Anaphylactic shock.

Multiple choice questions *(Answers to Q. 12–13 appear on pp. 180–181)*
Questions 12 and 13 are multiple choice questions.

---

12. Which one of the following drugs would most likely be given in the accident and emergency department to relieve Matthew's pain?
    A. Intravenous morphine sulphate
    B. Subcutaneous papaveretum (Omnopon)
    C. Intramuscular dihydrocodeine (D.F. 118)
    D. Oral pethidine hydrochloride.

13. Which one of the following pins would be inserted through Mattew's left tibial condyle in order to exert traction on his femur?
    A. Moore's pin
    B. Küntscher nail
    C. Steinmann's pin
    D. Garden nail.

Matthew's leg was placed on a Thomas' splint with a Pearson's flexion piece attached. The traction cord from the pin was passed over a pulley at the foot of the bed and the splint was suspended from the Balkan beam.

Matthew spent his first night in hospital in the intensive care unit.

True/false statements *(Answers to Q. 14–28 appear on pp. 182–185)*
The following questions (14–28) are true/false statements.

---

14. When selecting a Thomas' splint for Matthew, one with a buckle adjustment in the ring could be chosen.

15. In this type of traction, counter-traction is exerted by the pressure of the ring on the ischial tuberosity.

16. The fracture is reduced by gradually increasing the weight on the traction over a period of a few days.

17. A pad of wool should be placed behind the fracture site to maintain the correct position.

18. The lower leg should rest on the Pearson's flexion piece so that the knee is at an angle of 90°.

19. Matthew should be nursed sitting up with a back-rest and pillows to support him.

20. Matthew should be encouraged to lift himself up with the use of a pulley (Monkey pole).

The next morning Matthew's condition was much improved and he was transferred to the orthopaedic ward. Student Nurse Maxwell was allocated to care for him during the next few days when she was on duty. The ward sister pointed out the importance of caring for his skin, especially under the ring of the Thomas' splint, and also the need to check the traction daily.

Which of the following courses of action should Nurse Maxwell take to prevent pressure sores developing under the ring of the Thomas' splint? Answer true or false.

21. Push the splint up and down his leg every two hours.

22. Teach Matthew to move the skin under the ring.

23. Wash and dry the skin under the ring.

24. Place a clean piece of lint between the ring and the skin.

Which of the following should Nurse Maxwell do when checking and adjusting Matthew's traction daily? Again answer true or false.

25. Examine the skeletal pin site and cleanse if required.

26. Twist the skeletal pin to prevent it adhering to the bone.

27. Ensure that the cords are running smoothly over the pulleys.

28. Remove the weights if Matthew's bed is moved.

Matthew recovered quickly from his accident and within a few days he had settled well on his traction. Four days after his accident his leg was relatively pain-free and he commenced physiotherapy.

Six weeks later check X-rays of his femur showed that he had quite a large callus forming. The surgeon decided that his traction should be removed and a cast-brace was applied, and one week later he was discharged home.

Multiple choice questions *(Answers to Q. 29–30 appear on pp. 185–188)*
The following questions (29–30) are mutliple choice questions.

29. Which one of the following exercises should the physiotherapist *not* teach Matthew when he *begins* exercising his injured leg?
    A. Static quadriceps exercises
    B. Knee flexion exercises
    C. Plantarflexion and dorsiflexion of the foot
    D. Straight leg raising.

30. Which one of the following is *not* an advantage of the cast-brace in the treatment of a fractured shaft of femur.
    A. It allows movement of the joints above and below the fracture
    B. It enables the patient to be mobilized early
    C. It can be removed when the patient goes to bed
    D. It allows the patient to take weight on the injured leg.

Matthew made good progress at home and, eight weeks after it had been applied, the cast-brace was removed. X-rays and clinical examination showed that the fracture was well healed.

True/false statements *(Answers to Q. 31–44 appear on pp. 189–192)*
The following questions (31–36) are true/false statements about the healing of fractures.

31. Matthew's fracture is likely to unite quickly because it is a transverse fracture.

32. Callus is formed from the periosteum and from the marrow cavity.

33. Once a callus has formed the bone can be described as having united.

34. The site of a fracture will always be visible on X-ray.

35. Bony union of the fracture will not occur unless the fractured bones are immobilized.

36. Callus does not usually form when the fracture is rigidly held by internal metal fixation.

The following questions (37–44) are true/false statements about the complications of a fractured shaft of the femur. Again answer true or false.

37. Stiffness of the knee joint does not occur if the fracture has been treated by balanced traction.

38. Distraction of the fracture may lead to delayed union.

39. Sciatic nerve damage is rare in this type of fracture.

40. Fat embolism is a common complication of a fractured shaft of femur.

41. A fat embolus usually occurs 5 days after the injury.

42. A fat embolus is usually caused by globules of fat entering the blood circulation from damaged adipose tissue.

43. 14 weeks after the injury Matthew's fracture should be united well enough for him to walk without crutches.

44. Fractures of the shaft of the femur often refracture after the removal of the splintage.

Fractured shaft of femur answers

1. **C** The first-aider should first organize someone to stop oncoming traffic so that further injuries do not occur from a vehicle crashing into the scene of the accident on a wet, dark night. Matthew's injuries should then be evaluated (D) and an ambulance sent for (A).

2. **A** As the accident has occurred in the town centre, Matthew will probably be transferred to hospital quickly, so it would be inadvisable to attempt to move him. He should therefore be covered with a coat or blanket and made as comfortable as possible until the ambulance arrives (A). An inflatable splint could then be applied by the ambulance men who should take care not to over-inflate it as this can cause compression of the blood vessels and gangrene.

   If the accident had occurred in a country area, where there is likely to be some delay before the ambulance arrives, then his feet could have been tied together (B) or to a firm object like a broom handle (C) so that he could have been moved to a safer and more sheltered position. Care should be taken when immobilizing his legs not to move the fracture more than necessary as the fractured bone ends may damage blood vessels or nerves. It would probably be better not to remove his crash helmet (C) as he may have sustained head or neck injuries and the helmet would also serve to keep his head warm and dry and thus prevent heat loss. Because of the possibility of injury to his neck Matthew's head should be carefully supported whenever he is moved.

   Matthew should not be given whisky or anything else by mouth (D) as he may require an anaesthetic to reduce his fracture. In addition, whisky would increase the state of shock by causing dilatation of the peripheral blood vessels and thus counteracting nature's own response to injury. It should not be given if there is any possibility that a head injury has been sustained.

3. **D** By asking Matthew if he remembers the accident the first-aider can ascertain whether he has lost consciousness at any time. Any changes in his level of consciousness or his speech during the time when the first-aider is attending must be noted and the ambulance crew informed.

The other three questions are of less importance to the first-aider but the answers will be required by the hospital staff, especially if Matthew is to have an anaesthetic.

4. **C** Any person who is involved in an accident in which a licensed, and therefore insurable, vehicle is involved is liable to be charged a fee for the treatment at the accident and emergency department.

5. **D** Having first ascertained that Matthew is conscious and has a clear airway, the nurse should then record his pulse, blood pressure, temperature, level of consciousness and pupil reactions as a baseline. In view of the fact that Matthew has a graze on his forehead, head injury observations should be carried out even though there is no evidence that he lost consciousness.

Once the nurse is satisfied with his general state, all his details can be recorded, an identification band can be placed on his arm (A) and he can be undressed in preparation for the doctor's examination (B). There should be no need to check the resuscitation equipment when Matthew comes into the accident and emergency department as it should always be left ready for use (C).

6. **C**
7. **A**
8. **D**

Before a blood transfusion is given, the blood group of the patient should be identified and this should be cross-matched with the donor blood (i.e. to check compatibility). If cross-matching is incorrect, or incompatible blood is given, agglutination occurs (the clumping together of the recipient's red blood cells), and may cause death. Only in an emergency, where the patient's life is put at risk by waiting for these results, should blood be given before first cross-matching it.

It will be recalled that the factors involved in an *agglutination* reaction are an *agglutinogen* present on the donor's red blood cells and a specific *agglutinin* present in the recipient's plasma.

There are four main blood groups: O, A, B, AB.

O — which has *no agglutinogens* present on the red cells but has *anti-A and anti-B agglutinins* present in the plasma. A patient with this blood group can recieve only blood of group O.

A — which has the *agglutinogen A* present on the red cells and *anti-B agglutinin* in the plasma. A patient with this blood group could receive blood of groups A or O but not B or ΛB.

B — which has *agglutinogen B* present on the red cells and *anti-A agglutinin* in the plasma. A patient with this blood group can receive blood of groups B or O but not A or AB.

AB — which has the *agglutinogens A and B* present on the red cells but *no agglutinin* in the plasma. A patient with this blood group can receive blood from any of the other blood groups.

Blood group	Agglutinogen on cell	Agglutinin in plasma	Can receive blood of group
O	None	Anti-A and anti-B.	O only
A	A	Anti-B	A and O
B	B	Anti-A	B and O
AB	A and B	None	A, B, AB and O

Therefore, blood transfusions can be given along the lines indicated by the arrows.

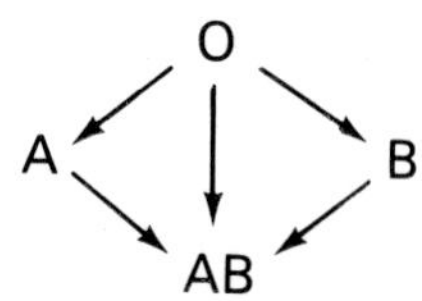

It can be seen that group O blood can be given to patients of any blood group. It is known as the 'universal donor'. Likewise, group AB is known as the 'universal recipient', as patients of this blood group can receive blood from any blood group.

There are other factors which may cause incompatibility, the most important of these is the *rhesus factor.* 85% of people have this antigen present in the red blood cells — they are classed as rhesus +ve (positive). The other 15% do not have it and they are classed as rhesus −ve, (negative). Should rhesus +ve blood be given to a person who is rhesus −ve, antibodies will be formed causing agglutination of the red cells. There is no such reaction if rhesus negative blood is given to a person who is rhesus positive. So a person who is rhesus positive can receive rhesus negative or rhesus positive blood.

From this we can see how the answers to questions 6, 7 and 8 are obtained. A person who is blood group A positive (Question 6) can receive blood of groups A or O and the blood could be rhesus negative or positive. Of the options given (C) is correct.

A person of blood group B negative (Question 7) could receive blood of groups B or O but the blood must be rhesus negative; therefore (A) is the correct answer.

A person with blood group O positive (Question 8) would only be able to receive blood of group O but as he is rhesus positive it could be either rhesus negative or positive. (D) is therefore the correct answer.

Should Matthew require a blood transfusion before his blood has been grouped and cross-matched the universal donor (O negative) would be given.

9. **A** Oligaemic shock is caused by severe blood loss where the actual volume of blood circulating is reduced. The bleeding may be external, as in a laceration of a major blood vessel, or internal, such as bleeding into the stomach as in a bleeding gastric ulcer, or the abdominal cavity as in a ruptured spleen.

Mild oligaemic shock occurs if 10 to 20% of the blood volume is lost. It is treated by restoring the blood volume with plasma or intravenous fluids. If 30% of the circulating blood volume is lost, severe shock occurs, requiring urgent replacement by blood transfusion. Unless the treatment of severe shock is prompt and adequate, irreversible shock will occur.

The signs of shock are falling blood pressure, rising pulse rate, cold clammy skin, clouding of consciousness, and vomiting. If treatment is not given or the haemorrhage is not stopped, the urinary output falls, unconsciousness develops, and finally death will occur.

10. **B** Fainting is an example of neurogenic shock, where the blood volume is unaltered but nervous stimulation, via the vagus nerve, causes dilatation of certain blood vessels. The vessels chiefly affected are the splanchnic (abdominal) vessels, and the result is the pooling of blood in them, which prevents adequate perfusion of the brain and the heart. The brain is thus deprived of oxygen and the person loses consciousness.

Causes of neurogenic shock include pain, fear, standing still in extreme heat or sunshine, or a horrific experience such as witnessing an accident.

In this type of shock the pulse rate is usually slow. The treatment is to lie the person down, loosen any tight clothing and allow adequate ventilation.

11. **D** Anaphylactic shock is the type of shock which follows the administration of a drug to which the patient is hypersensitive. The reaction may be mild or it may be very severe, leading to rapid death. It is treated by giving intravenous adrenalin to try to restore the normal vascular tone.

12. **A** Of the drugs listed, morphine sulphate is generally considered to be the most effective analgesia where shock is present. Because the peripheral circulation is poor it is best given by intravenous injection, or 10 mg may be given intravenously and 10 mg by intramuscular injection.

Papaveretum (B) contains anhydrous morphine 50% with other opium alkaloids. It is therefore less powerful than morphine — 10 mg of papaveretum is the equivalent in morphine content to 6.25 mg of morphine sulphate. If it were given by subcutaneous injection to a shocked patient it would not be dispersed around the body due to the poor peripheral circulation. Further doses or another drug might be given later because it was thought that the first dose had not been effective. The cumulative effect of these could result in a drug overdose when the patient's blood pressure returns to normal.

Dihydrocodeine (D.F.118) (C) is used for mild or moderate pain and is not generally considered to be suitable for the acute pain accompanied by shock from which Matthew would be suffering.

Oral pethidine hydrochloride (D) would not be prescribed because of the delay in absorption and the possibility that an anaesthetic might be required to reduce Matthew's fracture. Pethidine hydrochloride might be given by intravenous or intramuscular injection.

It must be stressed that all analgesics should be withheld if there is any evidence of a head injury or hidden abdominal injuries, as they may conceal changes in the mental state or internal bleeding. In addition, morphine has the effect of constricting the pupils.

13. **C** A Steinmann's or Denham pin is most commonly used for skeletal traction. It is usually inserted behind the tibial tuberosity and through the tibial condyles but is sometimes inserted through the femoral condyles.

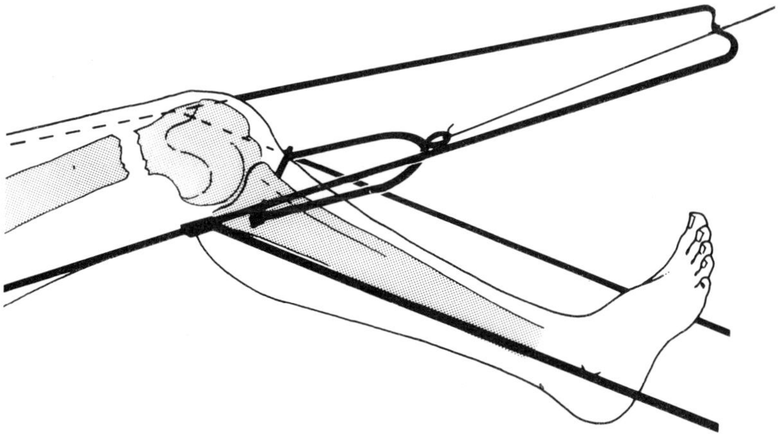

The position of a Steinmann's pin through the tibial condyle.

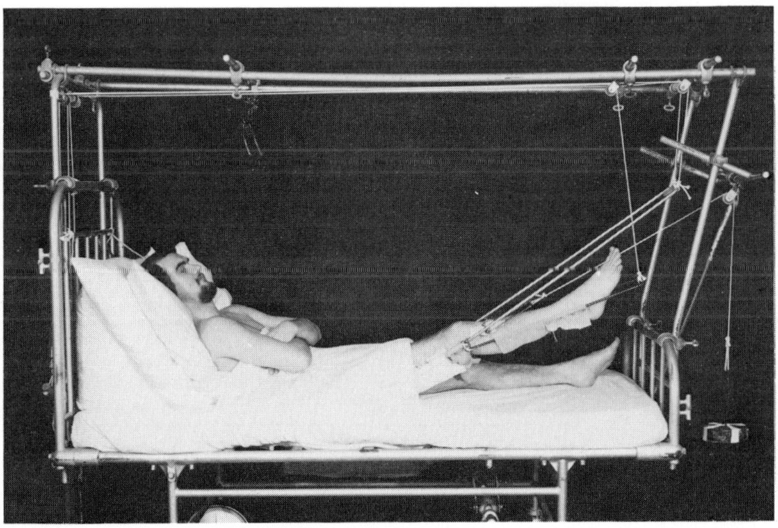

A patient on skeletal traction with a Thomas' splint and Pearson's flexion piece.

Note: the foot of the bed should be elevated.

Moore's pins (A) are used to reduce and hold a slipped upper femoral epiphysis; Küntscher nail (B) is an intermedullary nail used for immobilizing a fractured shaft of femur; and a Garden nail (D) is an internal device used in the treatment of a fractured neck of femur.

14. **True** Matthew's leg is likely to swell quite a bit during the next 48 hours. If a Thomas' splint with a buckle in the ring is used, the ring can be adjusted so that a constant snug fit can be maintained. An ill-fitting ring leads to pressure sores developing, so it is important that the splint fits correctly without being too tight or too slack.

15. **False** This is an example of balanced traction where the splint is used to suspend and support the leg. The foot of the bed must be elevated, and the weight of Matthew's body on an inclined plane will be the counter-traction. (For further details on the principles of traction and counter-traction, see answer 15 of Fractured neck of femur.)

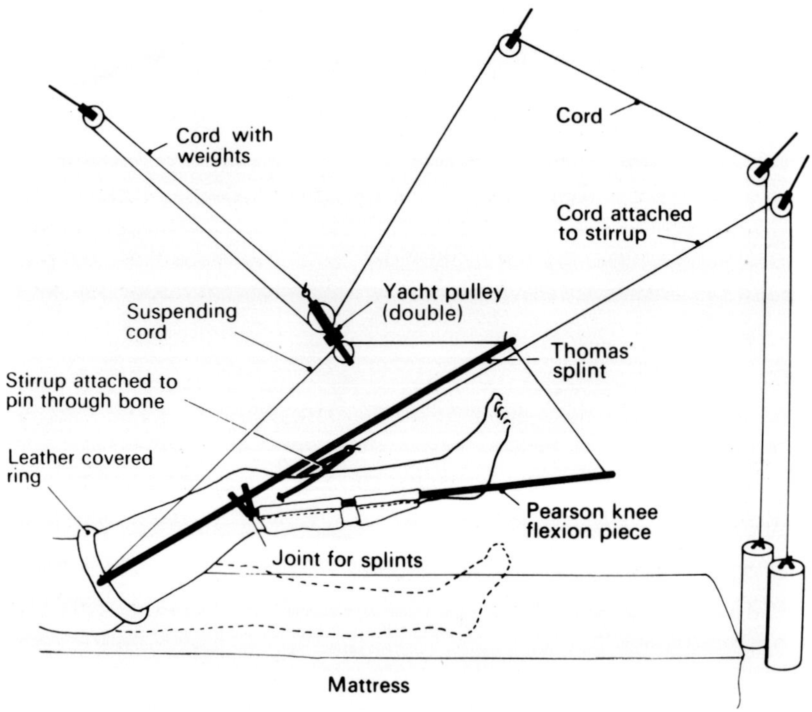

One method of suspending the Thomas' splint. Again the foot of the bed should be elevated.

16. **False** The fracture is reduced during the manipulation and the initial application of the splint. X-rays are taken to ensure that a satisfactory position has been achieved before the splint is finally bandaged into place.

Gradually increasing the weight and altering the position of the fracture can lead to delayed union or even non-union and should be avoided.

17. **True** In order to maintain the correct curvature of the femur it is necessary to place a firm pad, and sometimes a gutter splint, behind the fracture. Firm padding is needed behind the distal fragment to prevent backward displacement caused by the pull of the gastrocnemius muscle which has its origin on the lateral and medial condyles of the femur. This is particularly so in a fracture of the lower third of the femur.

18. **False** The Pearson flexion piece should be suspended from the overhead beam or from the end of the Thomas' splint so that the knee is at an angle of about 30°C.

19. **False** Sitting up with a back-rest would cause the ring of the splint to press into his groin. Until he has become accustomed to wearing the splint and the swelling of his thigh has subsided, he should be nursed in the semi-recumbent position with about three pillows to support him.

20. **True** Encouraging Matthew to lift himself with his pulley (monkey pole) will help the nurses when they are treating his pressure areas and enable him to relieve the pressure himself. In addition, it will strengthen his arms in preparation for the time when he starts to use his crutches.

21. **False** The splint should not be moved up and down in order to relieve the pressure as this could disturb the fracture and the padding supporting it.

22. **True** In order to relieve any pressure from the ring of the splint on the groin and around the thigh, Matthew should be taught to ease the skin up and down every two hours so that the actual point of pressure is changed. The splint must fit correctly because pressure will occur if the ring is too large or too small. If a Thomas' splint with an adjustable ring is used it can be made larger if Matthew's leg swells, and the size can be reduced as the swelling subsides. This ensures a constant snug fit and prevents the need to change the splint if swelling occurs.

The pressure will be relieved further by nursing Matthew in the semi-recumbent position.

23. **True** In addition to relieving the pressure under the ring of the splint, pressure sores will be prevented by keeping the skin clean and free from perspiration at all times. The skin should be washed regularly, dried thoroughly and dusted very lightly with powder. Applying too much powder or failing to dry the skin properly can lead to soreness.

The ring of the splint must also be kept clean and if it becomes soiled it should be washed and cleaned with saddle soap in order to keep it soft.

24. **False** Unless a sore develops which requires a dressing, nothing should be placed under the ring of the splint as this will only increase the pressure. The lint is also likely to wrinkle, which will result in sores developing. If the leather of the ring of the splint is kept clean it should be softer than any material such as lint or wool which might be inserted.

25. **True** The sites of entry of the skeletal pin should be examined daily for any signs of inflammation indicating infection. If it is necessary. these sites should be cleansed and dressings applied using sterile techniques.

Some surgeons prefer the pin tracts to be dressed daily while others prefer them to be left uncovered. The important point is that great care should be taken to avoid infection of the pin tracts, as this could lead to infection of the underlying bone and necessitate the discontinuation of the skeletal traction before the fracture has united.

26. **False** No attempt should be made to move the skeletal pin in the bone once it has been introduced. Movement of the pin will damage the scab which has developed around the pin at the point of entry and will allow organisms which are present on the exposed part of the pin to track along and cause an infection.

27. **True** As with all traction, a daily check should be made to ensure that the traction is being maintained on the limb. The splint should be examined to make sure that it is positioned correctly and the bandages should be removed and reapplied if necessary.

In order to maintain constant balanced traction and to allow Matthew to move up and down the bed, the cords must run freely over the pulleys. They should be checked to ensure that they are securely attached to the splint and to the skeletal pin.

28. **False** The weights should never be removed unless the surgeon orders it, otherwise the alignment of the fracture may be lost. Nurse Maxwell should check that the weights are hanging freely and are not resting on the bed or on anything else.

If Matthew's bed is moved, care must be taken to move it gently so that the weights do not swing about.

29. **B** As soon as Matthew is reasonably comfortable on his traction he should begin exercises to strengthen the muscles of his thigh and prevent knee stiffness. These are static quadriceps exercises (A) and straight leg raising exercises (D) which are done with the knee extended. Once the quadriceps muscle is strong it will act to support the fracture and it is *only then* that knee flexion exercises (B) are begun.

Dorsiflexion and plantarflexion of the feet (C) should commence at once and Matthew should be encouraged to pursue them vigorously in order to prevent deep vein thrombosis developing. Once he has recovered from the effects of the accident he should exercise his uninjured leg and his arms so that they are strong when he begins to mobilize.

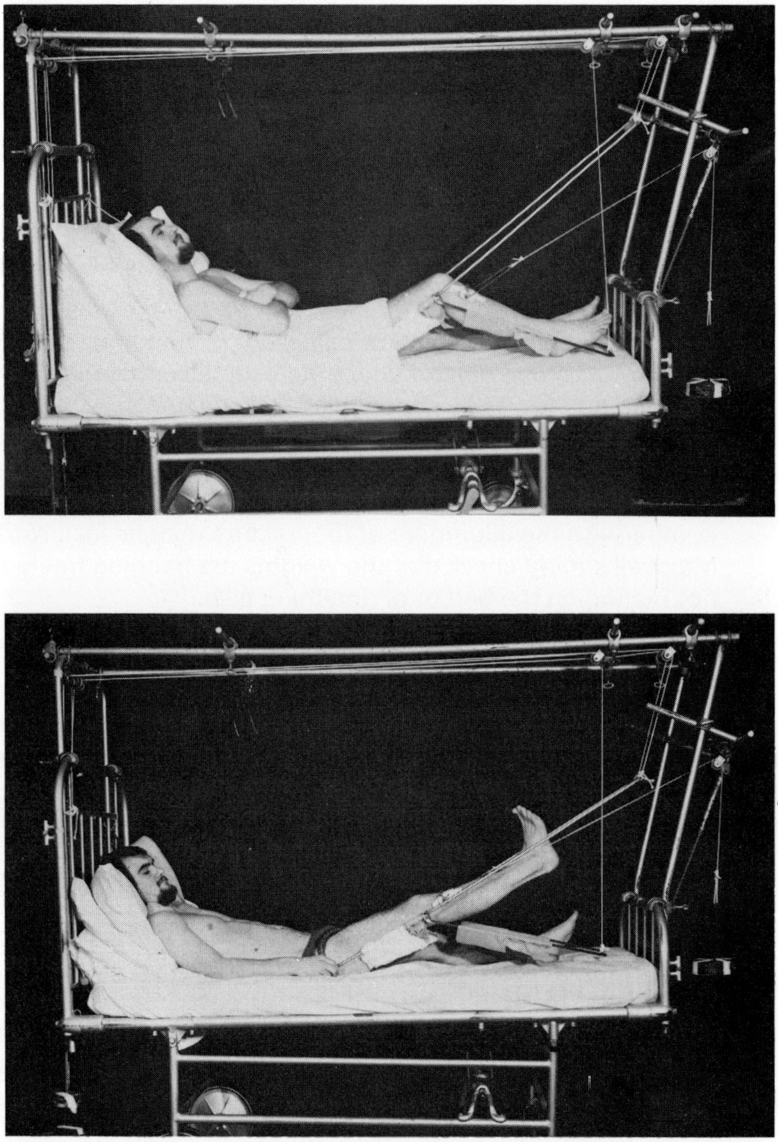

A patient carrying out flexion and extension exercises of his knee once his fracture has begun to unite.

30. **C** The cast-brace must be worn all the time. It is a functional brace which holds the fracture in the reduced position while allowing the patient to be ambulant and to take weight on the injured leg within weeks of the accident (B and D). In addition, the knee and hip are fully mobile which prevents joint stiffness from occurring (A).

The cast-brace consists of a closely moulded plaster of Paris applied to the thigh and a below-knee plaster of Paris which are connected at the knee joint by hinges. The above-knee plaster is applied over minimal padding and is carefully moulded to the contours of the muscle bulk of the thigh to give a quadrilateral total contact brace. The below-knee plaster is well fitting and may include the foot, or an ankle hinge may be inserted.

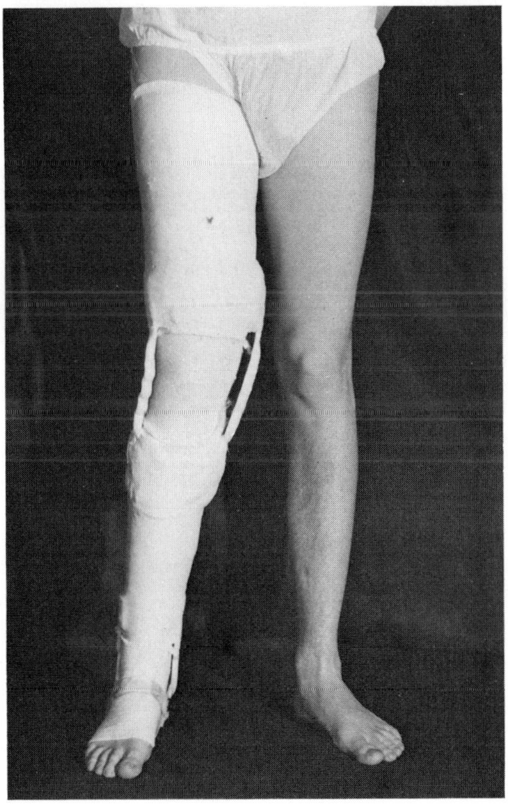

(a)

A cast brace with knee and ankle hinges.

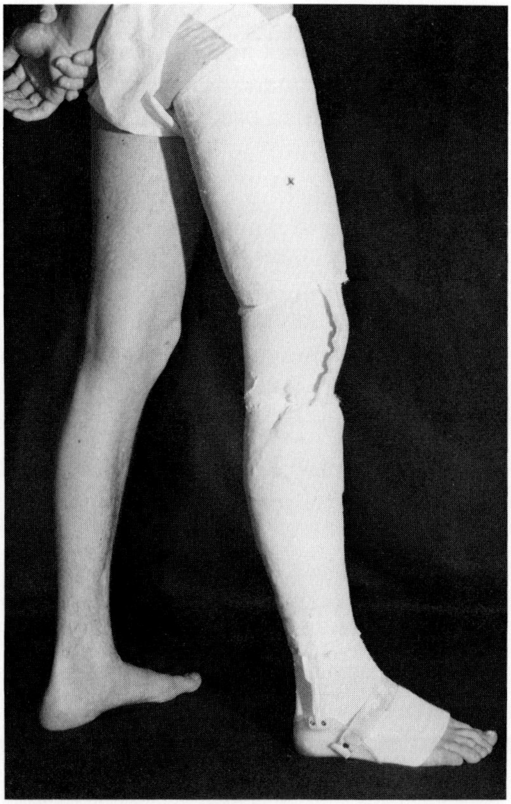

(b)

31. **False** Generally speaking, transverse fractures take longer to unite than oblique, spiral or comminuted fractures. This is because the area of contact between the fractured ends of the bone is smaller.

32. **True** An external callus is formed around the outside of the fractured bones from osteogenic cells of the periosteum. Osteogenic cells of the endosteum and bone marrow form the internal callus between the bone ends and the marrow cavity. Callus formation is the first stage of healing and it forms a bridge between the two fractured bone ends.

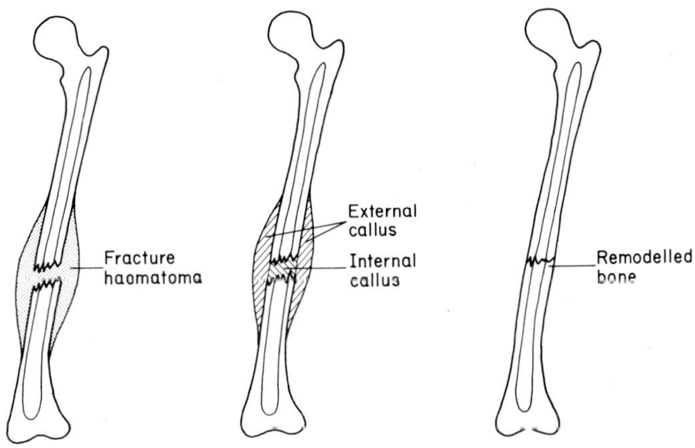

Stages of healing of a fracture.

33. **False** The fracture cannot be said to be completely united until consolidation has taken place. When this occurs, the callus is ossified and X-rays show the fracture line crossed by bony trabeculae. There is no tenderness or movement at the site of the fracture and the limb is now safe to be left unprotected.

The healing process of a fracture is a continuous one which begins at the time of the injury. When a bone fractures, blood vessels in the periosteum, haversian systems and marrow cavity are broken and a haematoma develops at the site of the fracture. This is known as the *fracture haematoma* and is formed by about 6 to 8 hours after the injury.

This haematoma is invaded by capillaries to form granulation tissue. Chondroblasts and osteoblasts are produced; the chondroblasts secrete phosphatase which stimulates the deposit of calcium, and the bridge of *callus* is formed.

Slowly the callus is invaded by bone cells (osteocytes), and it is replaced by a network of woven bone with trabeculae developing along the lines of stress. The immature bone is replaced by mature bone, pieces of dead bone are reabsorbed and the spongy bone around the edge of the fracture is replaced by compact bone.

34. **False** In adults the site of the fracture usually remains evident on X-ray for a long period, perhaps always, but in children the remodelling of the bone is usually more effective and the shape of the bone often returns to normal.

35. **False** Bones unite by producing callus which appears to be formed in response to movement at the site of the fracture. Many wild animals fracture bones which unite without any interference or immobilization. In order that they do unite, the fractured bone ends should come into contact with each other at some time so that the callus bridge can develop. The reason for immobilizing a fracture is to achieve union in the correct anatomical position and so give a good functional and cosmetic result. Immobilization also relieves pain.

36. **True** Experiments and clinical studies have shown that fractures which are rigidly fixed by metal so that no movement occurs at the fracture site do not produce the callus bridge. The healing still occurs by primary or direct union, where the osteoblasts and osteoclasts grow directly across the fracture with the bridge being formed by the metal.

It would appear that movement which occurs at the site of the fracture is directly responsible for the production of the callus: in fact the greater the movement the larger the callus. This type of union, where a callus is produced, is termed secondary or indirect union and is stronger than that produced by primary union.

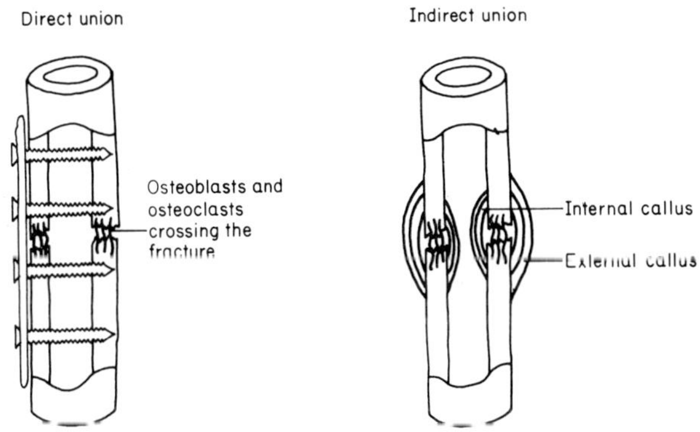

Direct and indirect union.

37. **False** Knee stiffness is less likely to occur with balanced traction than with fixed traction, but it could still be a problem if the knee is not exercised. The use of the cast-brace as part of the treatment further reduces the likelihood of its occurrence.

38. **True** Delayed union is particularly likely to occur in a transverse fracture if excessive weight is applied to the traction causing distraction of the fractured bone ends. This means that it is more difficult for the callus bridge to form.

39. **True** Because the bone is surrounded by large muscles, injury to the sciatic nerve or major blood vessels is not very common.

40. **True** Fat embolism occurs commonly in adults with fractures of the large long bones, although its clinical presence may be missed because the symptoms are so mild. It is only a small percentage who develop the serious signs of respiratory and systemic emboli.

41. **False** It usually occurs within the first 36 to 48 hours after the injury, and presents as a petechial rash particularly on the front and back of the chest, with a slight rise in temperature and pulse rate. In more serious cases the patient may be restless, dyspnoeic and may cough up blood. Unconsciousness could develop and finally death may occur.

Chest X-rays have a snowstorm appearance and right-sided heart failure may be seen on an electrocardiograph. Blood gases show hypoxia to be present, but the $_{p}Co_2$ is normal.

The treatment is to give O_2 to correct the hypoxia.

42. **False** It is very rare for a fat embolus to be caused by trauma to adipose tissue. More commonly, it is due to emulsified marrow fat from the fractured bone ends being forced into the venous channels within the bone. The fat then enters the general circulation.

43. **False** The safety of the fracture is not judged by the length of time since the injury but rather by the clinical stability of the fracture and the amount of mature bone seen on X-rays. Even if Matthew's fracture was found to be solid and pain – free on attempted movement, indicating that consolidation has taken place, it would be wise to give him crutches or two walking sticks for a short while in order to give the leg extra protection.

44. **True** Of all fractures, fractures of the shaft of the femur are the ones which most commonly refracture after the splintage has been discarded. The injury which causes this may be very minor, such as stumbling or tripping, and it usually occurs because the splintage has been removed before the uniting bone is strong enough to withstand sudden jerking movements. Bowing of the femur at the site of the fracture is sometimes seen and is due to weightbearing on the injured leg before the healing fracture is strong enough to withstand the strain.

Congenital dislocation of the hip

Thirty-two-year-old Janice Smithson is a dental nurse and her husband Tony is an English teacher at the local comprehensive school. When their first baby, Mandy, was born 10 months ago they were thrilled because they had wanted a child since their marriage 5 years ago. The birth was rather difficult because the baby was breech, but Janice soon forgot about that when she held Mandy in her arms. Mandy weighed 3.3 kg at birth and cried lustily.

The day after she was born the paediatrician examined the baby and found her to be completely normal except for her left hip which produced an audible 'click' on examination. The doctor explained to Janice that this might be due to a congenital dislocation of the hip and he arranged for an orthopaedic surgeon to see Mandy.

True/false statements *(Answers to Q. 1–14 appear on pp. 202–203)*
The following questions (1–14) are true/false statements relating to congenital dislocation of the hip.

1. Congenital dislocation of the hip occurs more commonly in boys than in girls.
2. It is more likely to occur in a baby whose mother had the condition at birth.
3. Babies born with the condition commonly demonstrate a general joint laxity.
4. Bilateral acetabular dysplasia may be present in a child with a unilateral dislocation of the hip.
5. The position of the baby in the uterus does not appear to be relevant to the condition.

6. The passage of the baby through the birth canal during a breech delivery may cause the hips to dislocate.
7. This condition is commoner in babies born to mothers over 40 years of age.
8. An amniocentesis would diagnose the condition during pregnancy.
9. Other congenital deformities may be associated with congenital dislocation of the hip.
10. It is more common for the right hip to be dislocated than the left.
11. There is a higher incidence of congenital dislocation of the hip in first-born babies.
12. There is a higher incidence in babies of Negro descent.
13. The hip dislocates posteriorly and laterally.
14. Accurate diagnosis is difficult until the baby is walking.

When she was three days old Mandy was examined by the orthopaedic surgeon and Janice was told that the baby's left hip was dislocated. She was measured for a Pavlik harness. Naturally Janice and Tony were upset by the news, but the surgeon spent time outlining the form that the treatment would take and reassuring them about the eventual outcome.

Matching item questions *(Answers to Q. 15–20 appear on p. 204)*
The following questions (15–20) are matching item questions relating to the pathology of congenital dislocation of the hip.

15–17 From the list on the left select the description of the pathology which is usually present in each anatomical part listed on the right.

A. Shallow and sloping	15. Neck of femur
B. Bony nucleus develops slowly	16. Head of femur
C. Retroverted	17. Acetabulum
D. Anteverted	
E. Small and flattened	

18–20 From the list on the left select the description of the pathological changes which occur in each part listed on the right if the dislocation is not corrected during infancy.

A. Atrophies	18. Capsule
B. Becomes large and folded	19. Labrum
C. Tears	20. Adductor muscle
D. Shortens	
E. Becomes hour-glass shaped	

Multiple choice questions *(Answers to Q. 21–26 appear on pp. 204–207)*
The following questions (21–26) are multiple choice questions.

---

21. Which of the following signs would indicate to the surgeon that Mandy has a congenital dislocation of the hip?
    A. Limitation of abduction of the left hip, asymmetrical thigh and buttock skin creases, and movement of the left leg causing distress to the baby
    B. Limited flexion of the hip, shortening of the left leg and a lump felt in the left buttocks
    C. Asymmetrical thigh and buttock skin creases, a lump felt in the left buttock and limited abduction of the left hip
    D. Shortening of the left leg, limited flexion of the left hip and movement of the left leg causing the baby distress.

22. Which of the following positive signs would indicate a congenital dislocation of the hip in a new-born baby?
    A. Trendelenburg and Ortolani
    B. Ortolani and Barlow
    C. Trendelenburg, Ortolani and Barlow
    D. Ortolani, Barlow and McMurray.

Mandy's Pavlik harness was applied 3 days later and Janice was taught how to care for her in her splint. She soon became confident in this and when Mandy was 10 days old they were discharged from hospital with instructions to return to the out-patients' clinic every week initially. Janice was told to bring Mandy back to the hospital at once if she was concerned about her or the splint.

---

23. Which one of the following is the position in which the baby's hip is held when a congenital dislocation is corrected?
    A. Flexion and abduction
    B. Extension and adduction
    C. Adduction and internal rotation
    D. Flexion and external rotation.

24. The chief advantage of the Pavlik harness is that it:
    A. Holds the baby's hips in one position
    B. Is easily removed for bathing the baby
    C. Allows the baby to flex and extend her knees while her hips are held in the correct position
    D. Allows the baby to kick her legs a little.

25. Which one of the following instructions would the sister give Janice when teaching her how to bath Mandy?
    A. Leave the splint in place and wash around it
    B. Remove one leg from the splint at a time for washing
    C. Take the splint off Mandy and bath her in the normal way
    D. Bath her in the baby bath with the splint in place.

Mandy continued with this treatment until she was six months old. X-rays and clinical examination then showed that a satisfactory reduction of the left hip had not been achieved and the surgeon explained to Janice and Tony that Mandy would need to be admitted for a period of traction after which a manipulation of the hip would be carried out. Arrangements were made for Janice to stay in the hospital with Mandy.

Two days after she was admitted, Mandy was placed onto overhead divarication traction (similar to Gallow's traction) with 0.5 kg of weight attached to each leg. After a few days the surgeon began to abduct her legs gradually.

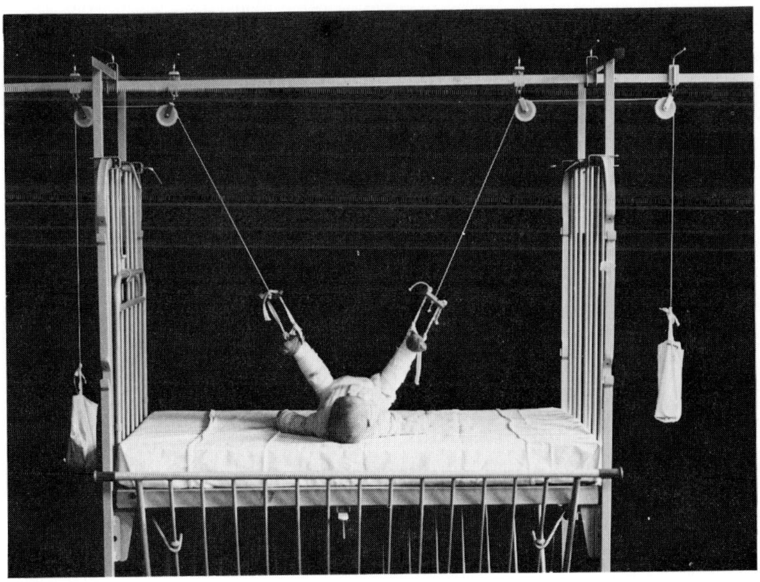

Baby on overhead divarication traction. (By kind permission from Downie PA 1984 Cash's Textbook of Orthopaedics and Rheumatology for Physiotherapists.)

During this time Janice was encouraged to care for Mandy with help and guidance from the nursing staff. She was allowed to nurse her on her knee at the bedside while the overhead traction was maintained, and always had her out of the cot for feeding. This was a great relief to Janice as she was still breast feeding Mandy and had dreaded not being able to nurse and cuddle her baby.

---

26. Regarding the X-rays, which one of the following statements is *not* true?
    A. A straight anterior-posterior film will show the dislocation
    B. Von Rosen's method of X-raying the baby's hips with the legs held at 90° of abduction will confirm the diagnosis
    C. Diagnosis can be confirmed with an arthrogram film
    D. A gap in Shenton's line indicates a dislocation.

True/false statements *(Answers to Q. 27–42 appear on pp. 207–210)*
The following questions (27–42) are true/false statements.

---

27. Before Mandy begins her traction she should have a zinc oxide patch test done.

28. The skin extensions should extend above the knees.

29. The aim of the overhead traction is to reduce the dislocation.

30. With this type of traction the weight attached to each leg is always 0.5 kg.

31. Janice should be taught how to care for Mandy's traction.

32. Constipation is often a problem in babies of this age who are immobilized on traction.

33. Janice should play games with Mandy which will encourage her to move around.

34. Mandy should wear a restrainer harness.

After three weeks of traction Mandy was given a general anaesthetic and an arthrogram was performed, followed by a closed reduction. A satisfactory correction of the dislocation was achieved and a double hip plaster of Paris spica was applied, extending from the nipple line to the toes, with the hips in flexion and internal rotation to maintain the position.

Her recovery from the anaesthetic was uneventful, and while her plaster was wet Mandy was turned 4 hourly. A wooden frame was made for her and when the plaster had dried she was nursed on this.

(a)

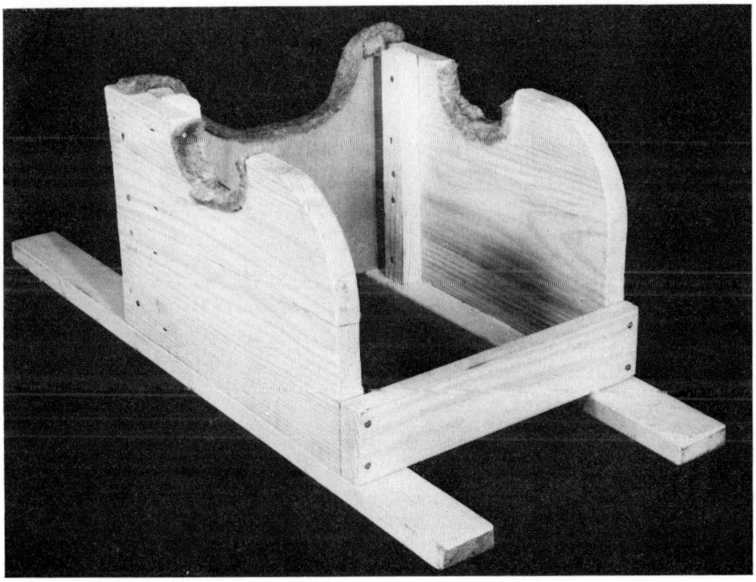

(a) A wooden frame for supporting a baby in a plaster hip spica. (b) A baby nursed on a wooden frame.

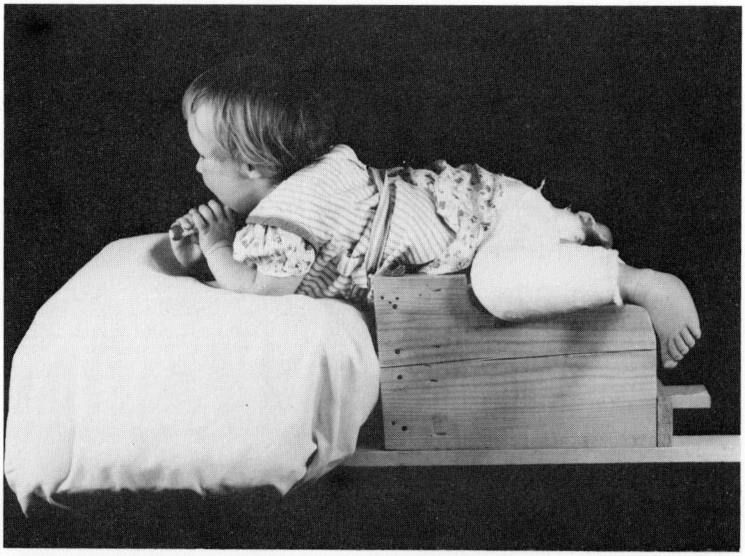
(b)

Janice was taught how to care for Mandy in the plaster and one week later she was able to take her home. Again she was told to bring her to the out-patients' department every week initially, and to contact the hospital at once should she have any problems.

---

35. The arthrogram is performed to confirm that the hip is still dislocated.

36. The hip spica should be applied with the knees in full extension.

37. Hip spicas applied in this way may restrict the baby's breathing.

38. A hole should be cut in the plaster over Mandy's abdomen as soon as possible after the plaster has been applied.

39. Vulval oedema frequently occurs in little girls after a closed reduction.

40. Until the plaster is dry and she can be placed on the wooden frame, Mandy should have a nappy to prevent her plaster becoming soaked with urine.

Two months later Mandy was re-admitted to the children's ward. Under a general anaesthetic her plaster of Paris was removed and her hip was examined. The surgeon found the hip to be in a satisfactory position but he did not consider that it was stable enough for her to go without a plaster hip spica. A new double hip spica was applied and, three days later, when the plaster had dried, Mandy was discharged from hospital.

Mandy has been home from hospital a month now and she returns to the clinic every two weeks. She is a very happy child and Janice has become quite confident about looking after her in the plaster. In another month she will be re-admitted and her plaster will be removed under a general anaesthetic. If her hip is considered to be stable she will probably have broomstick plasters applied for about three months and then, if all is well, she will begin mobilizing.

---

41. The day before Mandy's examination under a general anaesthetic the skin beneath the plaster should be examined and treated for soreness.

42. When Mandy is in the broomstick plasters she should be turned prone for a period each day.

Congenital dislocation of the hip — answers

1. **False** The incidence of congenital dislocation of the hip diagnosed at birth is higher in girls than boys with a ratio of 3:1.

2. **True** The causes of the condition are not fully understood and it is apparent that there are many contributing factors. There is evidence of a genetic factor associated with it, as a woman who had the condition as a baby is more likely to have a child with congenital dislocation of the hip than a woman who did not. This chance is further increased if the baby is female.

3. **True** This is thought to be due to a ligament-relaxing hormone being produced by the female fetal uterus in response to oestrogen and progesterone being absorbed into the fetal circulation. This may be the reason for a higher incidence of congenital dislocation of the hip in girls. In addition, one of the parents or a close relative may demonstrate joint laxity, indicating genetically determined hip instability, and this may be a determining factor.

4. **True** There is a high incidence of defective development of the acetabulum of both hips even when only one hip demonstrates a subluxation or dislocation. The cause of this dysplasia, and that of femoral head dysplasia, is usually genetic and is as common in boys as in girls. This, combined with joint laxity, may cause the joint to dislocate.

5. **False** A high proportion of babies born with congenital dislocation of the hip are born by breech delivery which indicates that there may also be a mechanical cause for the condition.

6. **False** There is no evidence to suggest that it is the breech delivery which causes the hip to dislocate, but rather the position of the fetus in the uterus, as a similar percentage of breech-presenting babies born by caesarean section also present with the condition.

7. **False** There is no evidence to suggest that the maternal age has any bearing on the condition.

8. **False** An amniocentesis can be performed to diagnose conditions where there are chromosomal abnormalities such as Down's syndrome, or when an abnormal protein is found in the amniotic fluid as in anencephaly or spina bifida. It has no value in the diagnosis of congenital conditions such as congenital dislocation of the hip.

9. **True** Other congenital deformities, such as congenital talipes equino-varus or congenital talipes calcaneo-valgus are associated with congenital dislocation of the hip. When these occur on the same side as the dislocated hip it suggests that uterine pressure may be the cause of the dislocation.

10. **False** Dislocations of the left hip are more common than those of the right and may be caused by compression of the left hip against the sacral promontory in a fetus lying in the breech position.

11. **True** 60% of babies born with congenital dislocation of the hip are first babies. The reason for this is thought to be the tight abdominal and uterine muscles commonly seen during first pregnancies, which prevent the fetus kicking and changing position in the uterus. A similar high incidence is associated with oligohydramnios (deficiency of amniotic fluid) where the fetal movement is restricted.

12. **False** There is evidence that the condition is common in certain areas of the world, notably Northern Italy and Japan, but it is fairly rare in Negro and Mongol races.

13. **True** The hip always dislocates posteriorly and the slope of the pelvis then pushes it laterally.

14. **False** It is standard procedure in the United Kingdom for all babies to have their hips examined at birth but, despite this, some cases of congenital dislocation of the hip are still missed. Early diagnosis and treatment is vital if the child is to be spared long periods of splintage and hospitalization. Delay in treatment may result in difficulty in reducing the dislocation and in damage to the hip and its supporting structures.

15. **D** In most cases of congenital dislocation of the hip the femoral neck is short and there is increased anteversion. The normal angle of anteversion between the femoral neck and the shaft in infants is 25°.

16. **B** In this condition the bony nucleus of the head of the femur appears late and it develops slowly. The cartilagenous head is often larger than normal.

17. **A** The acetabulum is underdeveloped laterally; as a result it is shallow and its upper surface slopes steeply instead of forming a horizontal roof.

18. **E** Unlike a traumatic dislocation, the capsule of the joint remains intact but, if the dislocation is untreated, it becomes increasingly elongated as the femoral head is displaced upwards. As time progresses, it becomes hour-glass shaped, with the narrow part compressed by the psoas muscle pressing against it.

19. **B** The labrum, which normally deepens the acetabulum, is often large and may be folded inwards. It is usually referred to as the limbus, and it can cause an obstruction when reduction of the hip is attempted.

20. **D** As time progresses, the adductor muscles arising from the pelvis become shortened. These shortened muscles, the constricted capsule and the inverted limbus may make reduction of a congenital dislocation of the hip which has been diagnosed late, difficult. Hypertrophy of the ligamentum teres, contracture of the transverse acetabular ligament and the presence of fatty tissue (pulvinar) in the acetabulum may all further hinder the reduction.

21. **C** On clinical examination, the thigh and buttock skin creases are frequently found to be asymmetrical in unilateral congenital dislocation of the hip. There is usually limitation of abduction of the affected hip, and the buttock on that side may be flattened. A lump, which is the head of the femur, is often felt in the gluteal region, and the affected leg may be shortened. Movement of the hip does not usually cause the baby pain.

22. **B** A baby's hip should abduct to 90° in flexion, but if the hip is dislocated it frequently stops at 45°. If the hip is pushed beyond this point an audible 'click' is heard. This is a positive Ortolani's sign and is present at birth. The 'click' becomes weaker after a few weeks.

Barlow's sign is similar but the examiner's fingers are held over the greater trochanters and the thumbs are pressed into the groins while the hips are abducted in flexion. This time an audible and palpable 'click' is felt if the hips are dislocated. Both these are diagnostic signs for congenital dislocation of the hip and all new-born babies should be tested.

Trendelenburg's sign is used when an older child is examined for congenital dislocation of the hip. In order to carry out this test the child must be able to stand. McMurray's sign is used when testing for a torn meniscus.

23. **A** The principle of the treatment of a new-born baby with congenital dislocation of the hip is holding the hip in flexion and abduction. In this position the head of the femur can be reduced into the acetabulum. One method of maintaining this position is the use of the Pavlik harness, but other splints, e.g. Craig nappy splint, Von Rosen or the Barlow splints, may be used.

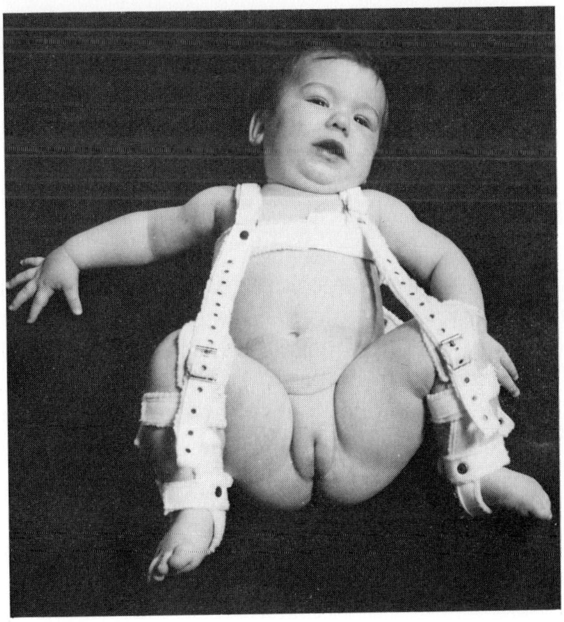

(a) Pavlic harness.

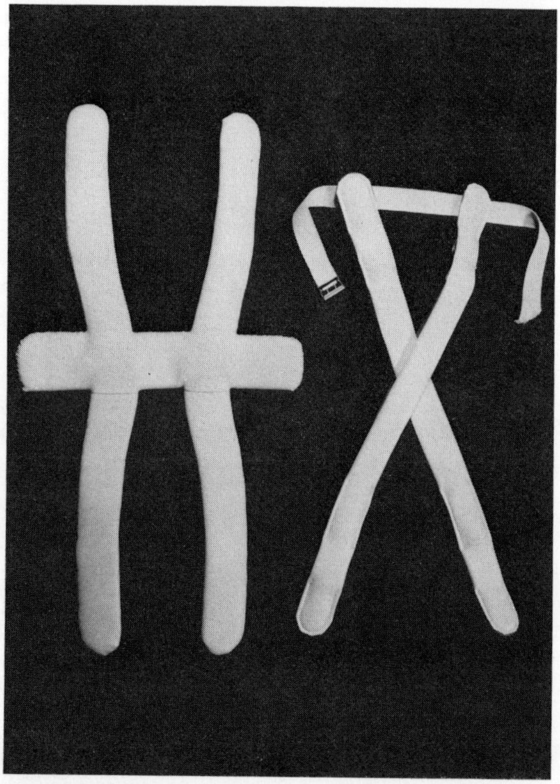

(b) Von Rosen splint (left) and Barlow splint (right).

24. D The chief advantage of the Pavlik harness is that the baby is able to kick its legs within the constraints of the harness. This spontaneous movement helps to achieve reduction of the joint. The Von Rosen splint and the Craig nappy splint do not allow any movement of the hip joints and may be used for a period before the Pavlik harness is used.

The methods of treating a baby with congenital dislocation of the hip varies from centre to centre. For further details of other methods of treatment it is suggested that the student studies other texts (see suggested reading list on p. 213).

25. **B** As the clinical evidence points to dislocation of the hip it is likely that Mandy should have one leg removed from the splint at a time for washing. When out of the splint the leg should be held in flexion and abduction, so it would be necessary for Janice and Tony to be taught how to bath her together — one holding the leg while the other washes it. The leg should be examined for signs of soreness, carefully dried and lightly powdered before being replaced into the splint. The other leg should then be washed in the same way.

If the clinical evidence had indicated a subluxation of the hip Janice and Tony would probably have been allowed to remove the splint and bath Mandy in the baby bath. Some splints, e.g. Von Rosen, can be worn in the bath but great care must be taken to dry the baby and the splint well afterwards.

26. **B** Von Rosen's method of X-raying the hips of a baby may be used to confirm the diagnosis, but when these X-rays are taken the legs should be held at 45° of abduction (not 90°) and are internally rotated. If the hip is dislocated the femur points to the ilium instead of the triradiate cartilage as in normal hips.

At the age of 6 months the nucleus of the head of the femur is usually sufficiently developed to show if the hip is dislocated (A). An arthrogram will give a clearer picture and may be performed to confirm the diagnosis or to establish if there are any soft tissues, e.g. a limbus or pulvinar, which are preventing the hip from being reduced (C).

Another method which may be used to establish that the hip is dislocated is to draw Shenton's line on a straight anterior-posterior X-ray film. This line is drawn along the superior border of the obturator foramen of the pelvis and continued along the medial border of the femoral neck. In a normal hip this line forms an even continuous arc, but when the hip is dislocated the line is interrupted (D).

27. **False** Extension kits for children are no longer made from zinc oxide based strapping so a zinc oxide patch test is not appropriate. However, as babies' skins are very sensitive, Mandy should have a patch test of the extension strapping to be used, although it is made from non-allergic material. Many centres still find it necessary to hand-make extensions for small babies in order to get a good fit.

28. **True** Long leg skin extensions are always applied. The traction would be exerted on the knee joints if below-knee extensions were used.

29. **False** With this type of traction the aim is primarily to stretch the soft tissues so that a closed manipulation can be carried out later without pressure or damage to the head of the femur. Other types of traction, e.g. the Wingfield frame or Alvik traction, may sometimes be used to reduce the dislocation.

30. **False** In order that the traction may be effective it is essential that the weight on Mandy's legs is sufficient to raise her buttocks just clear of the bed. The weight of her buttocks will then act as countertraction.

The weight attached to each of the baby's legs will therefore be adjusted according to the baby's weight.

31. **False** It is the nurse's responsibility to check and care for Mandy's traction, but Janice could be encouraged to help. The bandages should be removed daily and the skin should be examined for soreness and signs of any allergy to the skin extensions.

32. **False** Constipation is less of a problem in babies of this age on traction than it is in older children undergoing similar treatment. Mandy's diet should be the normal one for a 6-month-old baby and should include liquidized fresh fruit and vegetables which would prevent constipation. Janice should be told to give her extra fluids to drink, especially fresh fruit juices, to help keep her faeces soft, and this would also help prevent urinary tract infections. If constipation is not prevented by correct diet and adequate fluid intake, a mild laxative, such as half strength Dorbinex, may be required.

As Janice is able to hold Mandy on her knee for feeding, the problem of Mandy choking while being fed lying flat on her back is avoided.

33. **True** Janice should be encouraged to play with Mandy when she is awake. Games would stimulate her mentally, and also they can be devised to prevent complications occurring, such as joint stiffness.

Tickling Mandy's feet would encourage her to move them and so exercise the muscles of her calves and prevent ankle and toe stiffness. Toys and mobiles suspended above her cot would stimulate her to reach out, and in older children toys which, when grasped, play music or make a sound could be used.

34. **True** Most babies of this age wriggle about continuously when they are awake, so it is usually necessary, when they are on traction, for a restrainer harness to be applied. This will prevent them rolling over and over and getting tied up in the traction.

35. **False** The arthrogram would be performed to check that there is no structure, such as an inverted limbus or a pad of fat (pulvinar), preventing the hip from being reduced. If soft tissue obstructions were found, an open reduction would then most probably be performed.

36. **False** The double hip spica would be applied with the hips in the position in which they are most stable. This is usually in abduction and internal rotation with the knees held in a few degrees of flexion. Alternatively, a 'frog plaster' may be applied with the hips in full abduction and external rotation and the knees flexed to a right angle. It may be necessary to perform an adductor tenotomy during the manipulation in order to achieve the necessary abduction.

37. **True** Mandy's respirations would be shallow while she is anaesthetised. Unless allowances are made for this when the plaster is applied, it is likely to be tight when she wakes up and begins crying and breathing deeply. The nurses should observe for this during the first 24 hours and, if necessary, the plaster will need to be split.

38. **True** A 'blow hole' should be cut in the front of the plaster in order to allow for diaphragmatic breathing and to prevent pressure on Mandy's abdomen. This should be done as soon as possible after the plaster has been applied to prevent her vomiting.

39. **True** Vulval oedema, particularly on the side of the reduction, is common in little girls after a closed as well as an open reduction. Similarly, scrotal oedema occurs in little boys. When it occurs, the lower end of the perch should be elevated to aid the venous drainage and, if it is very severe, the nurse may apply cool saline soaks, taking care not to wet the plaster.

40. **False** For a little girl, a urinary collecting bag could be applied to collect the urine and so prevent the plaster of Paris becoming soaked with urine. Once she had been placed on the wooden frame, the urine could be collected in a potty placed under the frame.

41 **True** The day before Mandy is due to have her hip examined under a general anaesthetic her plaster of Paris should be bi-valved and, removing the front of the plaster first, the skin beneath should be cleansed and examined for any signs of soreness. The front of the plaster could be lined with plaster wool before being replaced. Mandy should then be turned prone and her back treated in the same way. Because a baby's skin is so delicate it is usually better to cleanse it with a baby lotion than with soap and water.

42. **True** Janice should be told to turn Mandy into the prone position for short periods each day. This change of position will encourage normal growth and muscular development, and will prevent renal and circulatory stasis. Tony could be shown how to make a low trolley on castors so that Mandy can get about the floor to explore and play.

Prolonged extension of the hip should be avoided as it may result in the hips dislocating. Janice should be told not to leave Mandy in the prone position for too long and to be careful not to over-extend the hip when she is turning her.

Bibliography

Prolapsed intervertebral disc

Apley A G, Solomon L 1982 Apley's systems of orthopaedics and fractures, 6th edn. Butterworths, London

Powell M 1986 Orthopaedic nursing and rehabilitation, 9th edn. Churchill Livingstone, Edinburgh

Warwick R, Williams P L 1980 Gray's Anatomy, 36th edn. Churchill Livingstone, Edinburgh

Osteoarthritis of the hip

Apley A G, Solomon L 1982 Apley's systems of orthopaedics and fractures, 6th edn. Butterworths, London

British National Formulary 1981

Powell M 1986 Orthopaedic nursing and rehabilitation, 9th edn. Churchill Livingstone, Edinburgh

Rheumatoid arthritis

Apley A G, Solomon L 1982 Apley's systems of orthopaedics and fractures, 6th edn. Butterworths, London

British National Formulary 1981

Golding D N 1979 Concise management of the common rheumatic disorders. John Wright and Sons, Bristol

Golding D N 1982 A synopsis of rheumatic diseases. John Wright and Sons, Bristol

Powell M 1986 Orthopaedic nursing and rehabilitation, 9th edn. Churchill Livingstone, Edinburgh

Fractured neck of femur

Adams J 1983 Outline of fractures including joint injuries, 8th edn. Churchill Livingstone, Edinburgh

Apley A G, Solomon L 1982 Apley's systems of orthopaedics and fractures, 6th edn. Butterworths, London

Powell M 1986 Orthopaedic nursing and rehabilitation, 9th edn. Churchill Livingstone, Edinburgh

Meniscectomy

Anthony C P, Thibodeau G A 1983 Textbook of anatomy and physiology. Mosby, St Louis

Apley A G, Solomon L 1982 Apley's systems of orthopaedics and fractures. Butterworths, London

Hughes S, Sweetman R 1980 Basis and practice of orthopaedics. Heinemann, London

Powell M 1986 Orthopaedic nursing and rehabilitation, 9th edn. Churchill Livingstone, Edinburgh

Ross J S, Wilson K J W 1981 Foundations of anatomy and physiology, 5th edn. Churchill Livingstone, Edinburgh

Colles' fracture

Apley A G, Solomon L 1982 Apley's systems of orthopaedics and fractures, 6th edn. Butterworths, London

Charnley J 1961 The closed treatment of common fractures, 3rd edn. Churchill Livingstone

Huckstep R L 1970 A simple guide to trauma. Livingstone, Edinburgh & London

Powell M 1986 Orthopaedic nursing and rehabilitation, 9th edn. Churchill Livingstone, Edinburgh

Fractured shaft of femur

Apley A G, Solomon L 1982 Apley's systems of orthopaedics and fractures, 6th edn. Butterworths, London

British National Formulary 1981

Nash D F E 1976 Principles and practice of surgery for nurses and allied professions, 6th edn. Arnold, London

Powell M 1986 Orthopaedic nursing and rehabilitation, 9th edn. Churchill Livingstone, Edinburgh

Congenital dislocation of the hip

Adams J C 1981 Outline of orthopaedics, 9th edn. Churchill Livingstone, Edinburgh

Apley A G, Solomon L 1982 Apley's systems of orthopaedics and fractures, 6th edn. Butterworths, London

Davies R W 1973 Heritable disorders in orthopaedic practice. Blackwell Scientific Publications, Oxford

Downie P A (ed) 1984 Cash's Textbook of orthopaedics and rheumatology for physiotherapists. Faber & Faber, London

Hughes S 1983 Aston's Short textbook of orthopaedics and trauma, 3rd edn. Hodder and Stoughton, London

Lloyd Roberts G C, Ratcliff A H C 1978 Hip disorders in children. Butterworths, London

Sharrard W J W 1971 Paediatric orthopaedics and fractures. Blackwell, Oxford